365 Homemade 30-Minute Quick Bread Recipes

(365 Homemade 30-Minute Quick Bread Recipes - Volume 1)

Vicky Johnson

Copyright: Published in the United States by Vicky Johnson/ © VICKY JOHNSON

Published on August, 12 2020

All rights reserved. No part of this publication may be reproduced, stored in retrieval system, copied in any form or by any means, electronic, mechanical, photocopying, recording or otherwise transmitted without written permission from the publisher. Please do not participate in or encourage piracy of this material in any way. You must not circulate this book in any format. VICKY JOHNSON does not control or direct users' actions and is not responsible for the information or content shared, harm and/or actions of the book readers.

In accordance with the U.S. Copyright Act of 1976, the scanning, uploading and electronic sharing of any part of this book without the permission of the publisher constitute unlawful piracy and theft of the author's intellectual property. If you would like to use material from the book (other than just simply for reviewing the book), prior permission must be obtained by contacting the author at author@jumbocookbook.com

Thank you for your support of the author's rights.

Content

365 AWESOME 30-MINUTE QUICK BREAD RECIPES 8

1. "amerikaner" (German Vanilla Biscuit) 8
2. 3 2 1 Muffins 8
3. 7 Up Biscuits 9
4. Absolutely Delicious Bran Muffins 9
5. Allergy Friendly Fruit Muffins (Wheat, Egg, Dairy Free) 10
6. Almond Apple Muffins 11
7. Almond Muffins Flourless 11
8. Apple Almond Muffins 12
9. Apple Date Muffins 12
10. Apple Muffins With Pecan Topping 13
11. Apple Oat Muffins 14
12. Apple Oat Raisin Muffins 14
13. Apple Spice Sour Cream Bran Muffins 15
14. Apple And Cinnamon Muffins (Vegan) 15
15. Apple Cheddar Scones 16
16. Apricot Oat Bran Muffins Low Fat 16
17. Arabic Honey Glazed Pistachio Muffins .. 17
18. Arctic Garden's Blueberry Muffins 17
19. Asiago Scones 18
20. Atlantic City Sour Cream Biscuits 18
21. Baker's Chocolatey Banana Muffins 19
22. Baking Powder Biscuit 19
23. Baking Powder Biscuits 20
24. Banana Biscuits 20
25. Banana Cinnamon Walnut Muffins 21
26. Banana Miracle Whip Muffins 21
27. Banana Muffins With Chocolate And Ginger 22
28. Banana Nut Chocolate Chip Scones 22
29. Banana Oat Bran Muffins 23
30. Banana Raisin Muffins 23
31. Banana Zucchini Chocolate Chip Muffins 24
32. Banana Oat Bran Muffins 24
33. Banana Praline Muffins 25
34. Bananaluscious Muffins 25
35. Basic Biscuit 26
36. Basic Carrot Muffins 26
37. Basic Cornbread 27
38. Basic Navajo Fry Bread 27
39. Beef And Cheese Biscuit With A Kick 28
40. Best Banana Bran Muffins 28
41. Best Cheese Cornbread 29
42. Best Ever Banana Muffins 29
43. Best Ever Eggless Banana Oatmeal Muffins 30
44. Best Scones 30
45. Better Cheddar Biscuits 31
46. Betty's Of York Tea Room Fat Rascals Fruit Buns/Scones 31
47. Bigfatmomma's Better For You Pumpkin Muffins 32
48. Bisquick Cinnamon Raisin Biscuits 33
49. Black Pepper And Bacon Drop Biscuits .. 33
50. Blackberry Scones 34
51. Blue Cornbread 34
52. Blueberry Cottage Cheese Muffins 35
53. Blueberry Doughnut Muffins 35
54. Blueberry English Scones 36
55. Blueberry Muffins Low Calorie 36
56. Blueberry Oat Bran Muffins 37
57. Blueberry And Lemon Muffins 37
58. Bran Muffins Low Cal 38
59. Breakfast Oatmeal Protein Muffins 38
60. Breakfast Potato Muffins #5FIX 39
61. British Yorkshire Pudding 39
62. BunnyLovingCook's Basic Easy Muffin Recipe 40
63. Butterscotch Pudding Muffins 40
64. Butterscotch Biscuits 41
65. Cajun Biscuits 41
66. Campfire Muffins 42
67. Cara Cara Orange Glazed Scones 42
68. Caramel Scones By June 43
69. Carrot Pineapple Muffins 43
70. Carrot Raisin Bran Muffins 44
71. Carrot And Bran Muffins 45
72. Carrot And Date Muffins Gluten Free 45
73. Carrot And Poppy Seed Muffins 46
74. Carver Brewing Company Raspberry Bran Muffins 46
75. Cheddar And Poppy Seed Potato Scones . 47
76. Cheddar Tarragon Cornbread 47
77. Cheese Oatcakes 48
78. Cheese Pecan Cocktail Biscuits 48
79. Cheesy Biscuits 49
80. Cheesy Treasure Muffins 49
81. Chef Boy I Be Illinois' Moist And Healthy

Cornbread 50
82. Chipotle Cheese Mini Muffins 50
83. Choco Low Fat Muffins 51
84. Chocolate Malted Muffins 51
85. Chocolate Ras Muffin 52
86. Chocolate Soy Low Carb Muffins 53
87. Chocolate Wattleseed Biscuits 53
88. Chocolate Zucchini Muffins 1 Point! 54
89. Cilantro Cheddar Drop Biscuits 54
90. Cinnamon Cornbread 54
91. Cinnamon Raisin Muffins 55
92. Cinnamon Raisin Scones 56
93. Cinnamon Scones 56
94. Cleaned Up Scottish Oatcakes 57
95. Coconut Flour Agave Nectar Muffins 58
96. Coconut And Raspberry Muffins 58
97. Coffee Muffins 58
98. Coffee Shop Cornbread Muffins 59
99. Corey's Biscuits 59
100. Corn 'n Blueberry Muffins 60
101. Corn Grits Cornbread 60
102. Cornbread Muffins 61
103. Cornbread And Basil Muffins With Fresh Corn 61
104. Cornmeal (Cornbread) Mix 62
105. Cracker Barrel Old Country Store Biscuits 63
106. Cran Bran Muffins 63
107. Cranberry Walnut Scones 64
108. Cranberry Zucchini Muffins 64
109. Cranberry Orange Muffins (Diabetic Friendly) 65
110. Crazy Biscuits 65
111. Crustless Breakfast Quiche Muffins 66
112. Custard Powder Biscuits (Cookies) 66
113. Dad's Breakfast Egg Muffins 67
114. Dainty Crusty Biscuits 67
115. Date Pineapple Breakfast Muffins 68
116. Deception Muffins 68
117. Delicious Low Fat/Low Cal Cornbread ... 69
118. Delicious Low Cal Banana Muffins :) 69
119. Double Apple Corn Muffins 70
120. Drop Biscuits 70
121. Dutch Oven Breakfast Biscuits 71
122. Easiest Muffins By Trisha Yearwood 71
123. Easiest Quickest (Low Cal) Pear (Any Fruit) Muffin For One 72

124. Easy Banana Choc Chip Mini Muffins 72
125. Easy Blue Cheese Biscuits 73
126. Easy Cheese Muffins 73
127. Easy English Scones 74
128. Easy French Onion Biscuits 74
129. Easy Herb Biscuits 75
130. Easy Low Fat Cornbread 75
131. Easy Sourdough Biscuits(Bisquick) 76
132. Eating Suburbia's Banana Oatmeal Scones 76
133. Elderberry Muffins 77
134. Even Healthier Morning Glory Muffins ... 77
135. Fat Free Banana Bread 78
136. Fat Free Cranberry Orange Muffins 78
137. Fat Free, Sugar Free Cholesterol Free Blueberry Muffins! 79
138. Fiber Rich Muffins 79
139. French Toast Scones 80
140. Fresh Tomato Biscuits 80
141. Fried Hot Water Cornbread 81
142. Fruit Filled Muffins 81
143. Gem Scones 82
144. Ginger Molasses Muffins 82
145. Gingernut Biscuits 83
146. Glazed Blueberry Biscuits 83
147. Gluten Free Casein Free Applesauce Muffins 84
148. Good Morning Muffins 84
149. Grandma's Best Scones 85
150. Great Biscuits 85
151. Grilled Egg Cheese And Bacon Biscuit 86
152. Ham Pineapple Pizza Muffins 86
153. Ham Or Sausage Cheese Muffins 86
154. Healthy Apricot Walnut Muffins 87
155. Healthy Banana Muffins 88
156. Healthy Banana Nut Muffins 88
157. Healthy Banana Oat Muffins 89
158. Healthy Banana And Chocolate Chip Muffins 89
159. Healthy Berry Muffins 90
160. Healthy Blueberry Muffins A Nigella Lawson Makeover 90
161. Healthy Blueberry Scones 91
162. Healthy Bran Muffins 91
163. Healthy Chocolate/Berry Muffins 92
164. Healthy Cottage Cheese Muffins 92
165. Healthy Ginger Carrot Muffins 93

166. Healthy Mystery Muffins 93
167. Healthy Prune Oatmeal Muffins 94
168. Healthy Spiced Butternut Squash Muffins 94
169. Healthy W.w Oatmeal Raisin Muffins 95
170. Healthy, Moist Bran Muffins 96
171. Hedgehog Biscuits 96
172. High Protein, High Fiber Blueberry Muffins 97
173. Holiday Gingerbread Muffins 97
174. Homemade Cornbread 98
175. Homemade Scones 98
176. Homestyle Biscuits 99
177. Honey Oat Biscuits 99
178. Honey Peach Bran Muffins 100
179. Honey Rice Muffins 100
180. Hot Water Cornbread 101
181. Ina's Cheddar Dill Scones 101
182. Italian Biscuits 102
183. Italian Garlic Biscuits 103
184. Jalapeno Cheddar Cornbread 103
185. Jane's Banana Chocolate Chip Muffins ... 103
186. Jay's Zero Cholesterol Light Muffins 104
187. Jelly Crystal Biscuits (Cookies) 104
188. Jen's Easy Apricot, Cream Ginger Scones 105
189. Jim N Nicks Cheese Biscuits 105
190. Joyce's Jiffy Corn Muffins 106
191. KFC Biscuits (Copycat) 106
192. Kim's Fat Free Mini Pumpkin Muffins ... 107
193. Kiwi Biscuits 107
194. Last Minute Gingerbread Muffins 108
195. Lemon Apple Oat Muffins 108
196. Lemon Cranberry Oat Scones 109
197. Lemon Muffins With Toasted Coconut Refreshingly Sweet! 110
198. Lemon And Mango Muffins 111
199. Lemonade Scones 111
200. Light Moist Rhubarb Muffins 112
201. Light And Fluffy Vegan Lemon Scones . 112
202. Lighter, But Scrumptious Oatmeal Raisin Muffins :) 113
203. Low Fat Banana Chocolate Chip Muffins 113
204. Low Fat Banana Muffins 114
205. Low Fat Banana Raisin French Toast 114
206. Low Fat Blueberry Muffins 115
207. Low Fat Bran Muffins 115

208. Low Fat Cheesy Spinach And Egg Muffins 116
209. Low Fat Mini Apple Crumble Muffins... 116
210. Low Fat Oatmeal Pumpkin Spice Muffins 117
211. Low Fat Oaty Apple Raspberry Muffins 117
212. Low Fat Yogurt Biscuits 118
213. Low Low Fat Best Blueberry Muffins 118
214. Low Cal Banana Bread 119
215. Low Fat Apple Orange Oat Bran Muffins 119
216. Low Fat Blueberry Scones (Using Heart Healthy Bisquick Mix) 120
217. Low Fat High Fiber Blueberry Bran Muffins 121
218. Low Fat Homemade Biscuits 121
219. Low Fat Oatmeal Pumpkin Muffins 122
220. Low Fat, High Fiber Orange Bran Muffins 122
221. Lower Fat Lemon Blueberry Scones 123
222. Lower Fat Raisin Bran Muffins 124
223. Malt O Meal's Magic Muffins (Sugar Free) 124
224. Mary's Oat Bran Muffins 125
225. Mary's Skillet Cornbread 125
226. Matthew's Healthy Low Fat Vegan Carrot Spice Muffins 126
227. Meg's Ham And Apple Biscuits 126
228. Mexican Bizcochitos (Crusty Sweet Biscuit) 127
229. Mimi's Banana Muffins 127
230. Mimi's Gingerbread Scones 128
231. Mini Cinnamon Raisin Muffins 128
232. Mini Ginger Scones 129
233. Mini Holiday Muffins 129
234. Miniature Mango Muffins 130
235. Miracle Carrot Muffins 130
236. Moist Cornbread Muffins 131
237. Moist And Healthy Banana Muffins 131
238. Mom T's Refrigerator Bran Muffins 132
239. Mom's Magic Muffins 133
240. Mom's Southern Homemade Simple Biscuits 133
241. Most Delicious Muffins 133
242. Muffins 134
243. Multi Grain Banana Muffins 135
244. Mushroom Egg Muffin 135

245. My Favorite Muffins 135
246. Nana Walnut Muffins 136
247. Nana's Walnut Biscuits 136
248. New England Blueberry Muffins 137
249. Non Fat Banana Muffins 137
250. Oat Biscuits 138
251. Oat Bran Applesauce Muffins 138
252. Oat Bran Blueberry Mini Muffins 139
253. Oat Bran Dinner Muffins 139
254. Oat Bran Muffins (And Variations) 140
255. Oatmeal Banana Muffins 140
256. Oatmeal Breakfast Muffins 141
257. Oatmeal Cranberry Scones 141
258. Oatmeal Drop Biscuits 142
259. Oatmeal Peanut Butter And Jelly Muffins 142
260. Oatmeal Zucchini Muffins 143
261. Oh So Yummy Peanut Butter Chocolate Chip Muffins 144
262. Oil Free Bran Muffins 144
263. Old Fashioned Baking Powder Biscuits .. 145
264. One Banana Bread Muffins 145
265. Only Bran Muffins 145
266. Oooey Gooey Incredibly Yummy Banana Cinnamon Toast 146
267. Orange Spiced Scones 147
268. Peanut Butter Bran Muffins 147
269. Peanut Butter Chocolate Chip Muffins ... 148
270. Pearl's Granola Muffins 148
271. Perfect Cornbread Muffins With Corn! .. 148
272. Pineapple Sweet Potato Muffins (Louisiana) 149
273. Pistachio Orange Cherry Craisin Scones With Apricot Honey Butter 150
274. Power Muffins 150
275. Pumpkin Applesauce Muffins 151
276. Pumpkin Bran Muffins 151
277. Pumpkin Granola Crumble Topped Muffins 152
278. Pumpkin Oatmeal Muffins 153
279. Pumpkin Whole Wheat Muffins 153
280. Pumpkin Oat Bran Muffins 154
281. Quick Easy Apple Muffins 155
282. Quick Applesauce Muffins 155
283. Quick Chive And Bacon Corn Muffins .. 156
284. Quick Jalapeno Cheddar Muffins 156
285. Quick Mini Monkey Breads 157

286. Quick Vegan Pumpkin Spice Scones With Flax Seeds 157
287. Quick Whipping Cream Biscuits 158
288. Quick Yogurt Scones 158
289. Quick Zucchini Carrot Muffins 158
290. Really Good Low Cal, Low Fat, Healthy Blueberry Oatmeal Muffins 159
291. Rice Krispies Muffins 159
292. Rosemary Garlic Buttery Biscuits 160
293. Rumford's Baking Powder Biscuits 160
294. Salba Banana Coconut Muffins 161
295. Salmon Orzo Salad And Cheesy Herb Muffins 161
296. Sausage Cheese English Muffins 162
297. Sausage, Egg Cheese Biscuits 163
298. Savory Breakfast Muffins. 163
299. Savory Cheese, Cranberry And Herb Mini Muffins 164
300. Savory Herb Biscuits (Sage And Caraway) With Garlic Butter 165
301. Scone Recipe (C.w.a.) 165
302. Scotch Pancakes Or Drop Scones 166
303. Season's Severed Finger Banana Muffins (Low Fat) 166
304. Self Rising Biscuits 167
305. Seriously Strong Scottish Cheese Scones 167
306. Simple And Scrumptious Banana Bread. 168
307. Simple, Healthy Pumpkin Muffins 168
308. Simple, Low Fat Banana Muffins 169
309. Six Week Muffins 169
310. Skillet Cornbread 170
311. Skinny Banana Blueberry Muffins 170
312. Snickerdoodle Muffins 171
313. Souper Cornbread 171
314. Southern Biscuits 172
315. Southern Cornbread Muffins 172
316. Southwest Biscuits 173
317. Special Banana Blueberry Muffins 173
318. Spicy Orange Bran Muffins 174
319. Strawberry Banana Wheat And Oat Muffins 174
320. Strawberry And Cream Cheese Filled Muffins 175
321. Strawberry Orange Muffins!!! 176
322. Sue's Rice Muffins 176
323. Sugar Free Cinnamon Raisin Muffins 177
324. Sumner's Favorite Healthy Rhubarb Scones

177	
325. Sun Dried Tomato Biscuits	178
326. Super Fast Easy Onion Cheese Muffins	178
327. Super Simple Cranberry Coconut Scones	179
328. Super Moist Cornbread	179
329. Sweet And Nutty Raisin Bran Muffins	179
330. The Best Peach Nectarine Muffins	180
331. The Realtor's Cheesy Pepper Scones	181
332. The Ruby Pear Tea Parlor's Cinnamon Chip Scones	181
333. Three Cheese Onion Muffins	182
334. Thunder Bay Grille Biscuits	182
335. Tims' Mom's Blueberry Muffins	183
336. Toasted English Muffins With Cheese	183
337. Uncle Bill's Yorkshire Pudding	184
338. Vanilla Freezer Biscuits (Cookies) (With Variations)	184
339. Vanilla Muffins	185
340. Vegan Apple Muffins	185
341. Vegan Carrot Ginger Muffins	186
342. Vegan Fat Free Biscuits	187
343. Vegan Tomato Rosemary Scones (With Gluten Free Option)	187
344. Vegetarian Pizza Muffins	188
345. Weight Watcher's Cheese Muffins	188
346. Wheaten Scones (Diabetic Friendly)	189
347. Whipping Cream Biscuits	189
348. White Chocolate Chip Macadamia Nut Scones	189
349. Whole Grain Blueberry Ful Muffins	190
350. Whole Grain Fruitcake Muffins	190
351. Whole Wheat Banana Flax Muffins	191
352. Whole Wheat Cottage Cheese Breakfast Muffins	191
353. Whole Wheat Cranberry Orange Muffins	192
354. Whole Wheat Honey Flax Biscuits	193
355. Whole Wheat Maple Muffins	193
356. Whole Wheat Oat Scones	194
357. Ww 1 Pt. Weight Watcher Muffins	194
358. Ww Instant Oatmeal Muffins (1 Ww Point Each)	195
359. Yo Yo Biscuits	195
360. Yoghurt Corn Muffins With Corn	196
361. Yogurt Banana Muffins	196
362. Yummy Chocolate Pumpkin Muffins	197
363. Yummy Healthy Muffins	197
364. Zucchini Lemon Muffins	198
365. Ice Cream Muffins	198

INDEX 199

CONCLUSION 203

365 Awesome 30-Minute Quick Bread Recipes

***

1. "amerikaner" (German Vanilla Biscuit)

Serving: 12 biscuits | Prep: 10mins | Ready in:

Ingredients

- 100 g butter, softened
- 100 g sugar
- 1 1/2 teaspoons ground vanilla
- 2 eggs
- 4 tablespoons milk
- 200 g flour
- 50 g starch (e.g.cornstarch)
- 2 teaspoons baking powder
- Icing
- 8 tablespoons icing sugar
- 1 lemon, juice of

Direction

- Preheat the oven to 180°C/350°F.
- In a big bowl cream butter, sugar and vanilla. Little by little add the milk and the eggs.
- In a second bowl mix flour, baking powder and starch. Add to the butter-mixture and stir in until just blended.
- Using 2 tablespoons drop 6 heaps of dough onto each paper-lined baking sheet (you will need 2). Make sure to leave enough space in between the heaps as dough will spread during baking.
- Bake for 15 minutes or until golden brown. Transfer to a wire-rack and allow to cool.
- If using the glaze stir together icing sugar and lemon juice and spread this onto the even side of the Amerikaner.
- Idea: For children you can spread the curved side of the biscuit with a chocolate icing and stick slivered almonds into them to make them appear like little hedgehogs. :).

Nutrition Information

- Calories: 233
- Sodium: 134.9
- Total Carbohydrate: 38
- Cholesterol: 49.5
- Protein: 3.1
- Total Fat: 7.9
- Saturated Fat: 4.7
- Fiber: 0.6
- Sugar: 24.2

2. 3 2 1 Muffins

Serving: 1 Muffin, 12 serving(s) | Prep: 5mins | Ready in:

Ingredients

- 3 ripe bananas
- 2 eggs
- 1 (15 1/4 ounce) box cake mix

Direction

- Preheat oven to 350 degrees. Mash up your ripe bananas in a mixing bowl. Add eggs and cake mix.
- Pour evenly into a muffin tin (sprayed with your favorite non-stick spray). Bake for approximately 22 minutes.
- You can use any cake mix - but I recommend Spice Cake, Yellow Cake or Chocolate Cake. Add chocolate chips and/or nuts if you like. Easy and good! I like that you don't need any

oil for this recipe. You can make 12 larger muffins (fill each 3/4 full) or 18 smaller muffins (fill each half-way).

Nutrition Information

- Calories: 192.8
- Sugar: 23.4
- Total Carbohydrate: 35.1
- Cholesterol: 31
- Protein: 3
- Total Fat: 4.8
- Saturated Fat: 0.9
- Sodium: 253.2
- Fiber: 1.1

3. 7 Up Biscuits

Serving: 9 Medium biscuits | Prep: 15mins | Ready in:

Ingredients

- 2 cups baking mix (Jiffy or Bisquick)
- 1/2 cup sour cream
- 1/2 cup 7-Up soda or 1/2 cup Sprite
- 1/2 cup melted butter

Direction

- Preheat oven to 450 degrees.
- Cut the sour cream into your biscuit mix. "Cutting in" is simply incorporating your sour cream, butter or shortening into your dry baking mix without using a mixer. You can use a fork, knife, pastry cutter or the tools God gave you, your fingers. You just want to make sure that each portion of your {wet} ingredient gets coated with the dry mix.
- Stir in 1/2 cup 7 Up (any clear carbonated drink will work). The dough will be very soft, don't worry.
- Sprinkle additional baking mix on to your counter, about a 1/2 cup seems to work just fine.
- Knead and fold dough until covered in your baking mix. Pat dough out, (no rolling pin needed) and cut biscuits using a round biscuit/cookie cutter. Don't have one, no problem, you can certainly use a glass or empty soup can to cut out your biscuits.
- Melt butter in a 9 inch square pan. I stick my pan and butter in the oven for a few minutes to melt the butter. Just a few though, the butter will burn, so watch it.
- Place cut biscuits on top of melted butter and bake for 12-15 minutes or until brown.

Nutrition Information

- Calories: 242.3
- Total Fat: 17.1
- Saturated Fat: 9.1
- Sodium: 389.4
- Fiber: 0.6
- Sugar: 5
- Total Carbohydrate: 19.8
- Cholesterol: 34.3
- Protein: 2.6

4. Absolutely Delicious Bran Muffins

Serving: 40 large muffins, 40 serving(s) | Prep: 10mins | Ready in:

Ingredients

- 3 cups Fiber One cereal (or All Bran)
- 1 cup boiling water
- 1 cup sugar
- 3/4 cup applesauce
- 1/2 cup egg substitute
- 2 1/2 cups whole wheat flour
- 2 1/2 teaspoons baking soda
- 1/2 teaspoon salt
- 2 cups skim milk, mixed with
- 2 tablespoons lemon juice

Direction

- Pour boiling water over cereal and let stand.
- Mix together remaining ingredients then add softened cereal.
- Bake as many as you'd like in muffin tins sprayed with cooking spray.
- Bake for 15-20 minutes at 400°F.
- This recipe makes 40 large muffins, and the batter will keep in the refrigerator for up to three weeks, so you can have fresh, hot muffins anytime!
- Enjoy!

Nutrition Information

- Calories: 64.1
- Fiber: 3
- Cholesterol: 0.2
- Protein: 2.1
- Total Fat: 0.4
- Saturated Fat: 0.1
- Sodium: 138.5
- Sugar: 5.1
- Total Carbohydrate: 15.9

5. Allergy Friendly Fruit Muffins (Wheat, Egg, Dairy Free)

Serving: 12-24 muffins, 12 serving(s) | Prep: 5mins | Ready in:

Ingredients

- Dry Ingredients
- 2 1/3 cups spelt flour (I use Bob's Red Mill)
- 1/3 cup sugar (your choice of natural or white, for sweeter muffins use up to 2/3 cup sugar)
- 1/2 cup potato starch
- 4 teaspoons potato starch or 4 teaspoons tapioca starch or 4 teaspoons commercial egg substitute
- 4 teaspoons cinnamon
- 2 teaspoons soy lecithin, powder . (I use Bob's Red Mill, NOTE (If you are allergic to soy, substitute 2 tsp of oil for this ingredient)
- 2 teaspoons baking powder
- 1 teaspoon baking soda
- 1/2 teaspoon salt
- 1/2 teaspoon xanthan gum (I use Bob's Red Mill)
- Wet Ingredients
- 2/3 cup coconut oil (I use Tropical Traditions and sometimes use 1/3 cup coconut oil and 1/3 cup coconut creme for added)
- 1/2 cup apple juice
- 1/2 cup applesauce
- 1/4 cup water
- 1/4 cup agave nectar (maple syrup, honey and brown rice syrup are all good substitutes)
- 1 teaspoon vanilla extract
- 1 cup apple, diced small

Direction

- Preheat oven to 350°F.
- Sift dry ingredients together. (This is important since the soy lecithin can clump).
- Whiz wet ingredients in the food processor until combined, alternatively, use a stand mixer with whisk attachment.
- Tip the sifted dry ingredients into the food processor or mixer bowl (switch to paddle attachment) and pulse or mix for a few seconds until just (really, just) combined.
- Add apples and mix again until just combined. (Mixing too long will make these tender muffins a bit dense). The batter shouldn't be stiff, but definitely is not a wet batter.
- Spoon batter into foil muffin liners; will make 24 mini muffins or 12 regular size muffins. (If using a muffin tin, grease it lightly first).
- Bake mini muffins for 22-25 minutes, and regular muffins for 35-38 minutes.
- If you used a muffin pan, let the muffins cool for a few minutes in the pan before tipping them out onto a wire cooling rack. Muffins made in the foil liners can be transferred to a rack right away.
- Enjoy!

Nutrition Information

- Calories: 175.5
- Total Fat: 12.2
- Saturated Fat: 10.5
- Sodium: 270.4
- Fiber: 1.3
- Sugar: 8
- Total Carbohydrate: 17.7
- Protein: 0.6
- Cholesterol: 0

6. Almond Apple Muffins

Serving: 10 muffins | Prep: 10mins | Ready in:

Ingredients

- 2 cups almond flour (almond meal)
- 3 eggs
- 2 tablespoons melted grass-fed butter
- 2 tablespoons honey
- 2 teaspoons ground cinnamon
- 1 -2 apple, cored and chopped in blender
- 1 teaspoon baking soda
- 1 pinch salt

Direction

- Preheat oven to 325 degrees, then core an apple. Blend apple(s) until finely chopped, but not pureed. Mix all ingredients together in a bowl, then fill muffin cups until 3/4 full. Bake for 20 minutes. Makes around 10 muffins, depending on size.
- I usually make these muffins on a Sunday, then have then on hand throughout the week. I use around two tablespoons of honey for mine, though this creates a semi-savory muffin. If you like your muffins on the sweet side, then use more honey.
- I use the butter from grass-fed cows in mine, but if you'd like to avoid dairy entirely, then two to three tablespoons of melted coconut oil would be a fine substitute. Also, the amount of apples you use depends on the size and taste. I typically use one large apple. I also slightly undercook mine (a toothpick doesn't come out completely clean) because I find that they get a little dry if cooked through. If you prefer a drier muffin, then cook around 23 minutes.

Nutrition Information

- Calories: 65.3
- Fiber: 0.7
- Cholesterol: 61.9
- Total Carbohydrate: 6.5
- Protein: 2
- Total Fat: 3.8
- Saturated Fat: 1.9
- Sodium: 183.3
- Sugar: 5.4

7. Almond Muffins Flourless

Serving: 6 muffins | Prep: 5mins | Ready in:

Ingredients

- 1 1/2 cups raw almonds or 1 1/2 cups pecans or 1 1/2 cups walnuts
- 1/4 cup pure grade b maple syrup
- 3 eggs
- 1 teaspoon vanilla extract
- 1/4 teaspoon sea salt

Direction

- Preheat oven to 375 degrees.
- In a blender, grind almonds until flour like, use a spatula to scrape down sides if needed.
- Combine maple syrup, eggs, vanilla and salt in a small bowl and mix well.
- While blender is running, slowly pour the mixture inches.
- Continue to blend until well combined.

- Pour into buttered muffin pan.
- Bake 11 minutes, until golden brown.

Nutrition Information

- Calories: 279.8
- Saturated Fat: 2.2
- Sodium: 250.1
- Fiber: 4.1
- Sugar: 10
- Total Carbohydrate: 15.9
- Total Fat: 20.7
- Cholesterol: 105.8
- Protein: 10.8

8. Apple Almond Muffins

Serving: 12 muffins, 12 serving(s) | Prep: 5mins | Ready in:

Ingredients

- 1/2 cup almond flour or 1/2 cup almond meal
- 1 cup all-purpose white flour or 1 cup all-purpose whole wheat flour
- 1/2 cup granulated sugar
- 2 teaspoons baking powder
- 1/4 teaspoon salt
- 2 teaspoons ground cinnamon
- 1/2 teaspoon ground cardamom (optional)
- 1/2 cup milk
- 1 large egg
- 1/3 cup applesauce
- 1 medium apple, finely chopped
- 1/3 cup almonds, finely chopped (optional)
- Optional Crunch Topping
- 4 tablespoons brown sugar (optional)
- 1 teaspoon ground cinnamon (optional)
- 2 tablespoons almonds, finely chopped (optional)

Direction

- Preheat oven to 350. Grease or line a 12 muffin tin.
- Whisk the flours, sugar, baking powder, salt, and spices in a medium bowl.
- In a small bowl, whisk the milk and egg until beaten. Add the applesauce and mix to combine.
- Pour wet ingredients into dry. Add the chopped apples and optional nuts and stir to combine.
- Pour batter into muffin tins.
- Mix crunch topping ingredients in a small bowl and sprinkle topping over unbaked muffins.
- Bake for 20-25 minutes, until cooked through.

Nutrition Information

- Calories: 95.5
- Sodium: 122.2
- Sugar: 9.6
- Total Carbohydrate: 20.3
- Cholesterol: 19.1
- Protein: 2
- Total Fat: 0.9
- Saturated Fat: 0.4
- Fiber: 0.8

9. Apple Date Muffins

Serving: 12 muffins, 12 serving(s) | Prep: 10mins | Ready in:

Ingredients

- 3/4 cup whole wheat flour
- 1 cup all-purpose flour
- 1 cup wheat bran
- 1 teaspoon baking powder
- 1 teaspoon baking soda
- 1 teaspoon cinnamon
- 1/3 cup dates, chopped
- 1/4 cup egg substitute (Egg Beaters)
- 1/4 cup brown sugar, packed

- 2 tablespoons vegetable oil
- 1 cup 1% low-fat milk
- 1 cup apple, peeled grated

Direction

- Preheat oven to 375°F.
- In a lg bowl combine the whole wheat and all-purpose flours, bran, baking powder, baking soda and cinnamon. Stir in the dates.
- In another bowl, beat the egg substitute with sugar and oil until well mixed, then stir in the milk and apple.
- Pour into the flour mixture and stir just enough to moisten, being careful not to overmix.
- Spoon into nonstick or paper-lined medium muffin tins, filling almost to the top.
- Bake in the preheated 375°F oven for about 20 minute or until firm to the touch.

Nutrition Information

- Calories: 144.1
- Protein: 4.3
- Saturated Fat: 0.5
- Sodium: 156.1
- Fiber: 4
- Total Fat: 3.1
- Sugar: 9.8
- Total Carbohydrate: 27.4
- Cholesterol: 1.1

10. Apple Muffins With Pecan Topping

Serving: 12 Muffins | Prep: 10mins | Ready in:

Ingredients

- 350 g plain flour
- 25 g butter
- 50 g dark muscovado sugar
- 50 g pecans, chopped
- 2 teaspoons baking powder
- 1/2 teaspoon bicarbonate of soda
- 1 teaspoon cinnamon
- 284 ml sour cream
- 1 egg, beaten
- 3 apples
- 2 -3 tablespoons milk

Direction

- Heat oven to 200c/gas 6. Line a muffin tin with cases. In a small bowl, use your fingers to rub 50gs of the flour together with the butter to make fine crumbs. Stir through 1 tbsp. sugar the chopped pecans, then set aside.
- In a large bowl, sift together the remaining flour, baking powder, bicarbonate of soda a pinch of salt, then stir in the sugar cinnamon set aside. Coarsely grate 2 of the apples, then beat together with the soured cream egg 2 tbsp. milk. Make a well in the dried ingredients quickly fold through the wet ingredients, adding an extra tbsp. of milk if really dry. Don't over mix or your muffins will be tough. It doesn't matter if there are lumps of flour.
- Spoon the mixture into the muffin cases- they should be about two-thirds full -then sprinkle over the pecan topping. Thinly slice the final apple, the poke slices into the tops of the muffins. Bake for 20 mins or until risen, golden a skewer inserted into the centre comes out clean.

Nutrition Information

- Calories: 260.9
- Saturated Fat: 4.2
- Sugar: 7.9
- Total Carbohydrate: 38.5
- Protein: 5.5
- Total Fat: 9.8
- Sodium: 145.2
- Fiber: 2.3
- Cholesterol: 31.2

11. Apple Oat Muffins

Serving: 30 mini-muffins, 10 serving(s) | Prep: 15mins | Ready in:

Ingredients

- 2 cups about 3/4 pound mcintosh apples, peeled and shredded
- 1 1/2 cups flour
- 1 cup quick-cooking oats
- 2/3 cup brown sugar
- 1 1/2 teaspoons baking powder
- 1/2 teaspoon baking soda
- 1/2 teaspoon salt
- 1/2 teaspoon ground cinnamon
- 1/4 cup nonfat milk
- 2 tablespoons vegetable oil
- 1 teaspoon vanilla extract
- 1 (8 ounce) carton plain low-fat yogurt
- 1 egg

Direction

- Preheat oven to 400 degrees. Coat muffin tin with cooking spray.
- Place apples on paper towels and squeeze until barely moist. Set aside.
- Combine flour and next 6 ingredients in a medium bowl; stir with a whisk Make a well in the center of mixture.
- In another bowl, whisk together milk, oil, vanilla, yogurt, and egg. Add to well of flour mixture, stirring just until moist.
- Stir in apples. Spoon batter in muffin cups. Bake for 8-10 minutes or until muffins spring back when touched lightly in center. Remove muffins immediately and cool on wire rack.

Nutrition Information

- Calories: 217.1
- Saturated Fat: 0.9
- Sugar: 18.9
- Total Carbohydrate: 39.9
- Cholesterol: 20.1
- Total Fat: 4.3
- Sodium: 264.4
- Fiber: 2
- Protein: 5.1

12. Apple Oat Raisin Muffins

Serving: 24 Muffins, 24 serving(s) | Prep: 10mins | Ready in:

Ingredients

- 2 1/2 cups plain flour
- 2 teaspoons baking powder
- 1 cup brown sugar
- 1/2 teaspoon salt
- 1 cup quick oats (not instant)
- 1 (425 g) can pie apples, mashed (apple sauce would probably do)
- 2 tablespoons smooth peanut butter
- 1/2 cup canola margarine, melted (or substitute)
- 1 cup skim milk
- 2 teaspoons vanilla essence
- 1 cup raisins
- 2 eggs

Direction

- Preheat the oven to 350 F (180 C).
- Stir dry ingredients together.
- Add apples and peanut butter to the mix.
- Mix the melted margarine with milk, eggs, vanilla and raisins.
- Pour into the dry mix and stir well, but just enough.
- Spoon into greased muffin tins.
- Bake for about 20 minutes.
- Cool on wire racks.
- Makes 24 medium size muffins.

Nutrition Information

- Calories: 141.5
- Saturated Fat: 0.3
- Sugar: 14.6
- Total Carbohydrate: 29.4
- Protein: 3.3
- Total Fat: 1.5
- Sodium: 100.7
- Fiber: 1.4
- Cholesterol: 15.7

13. Apple Spice Sour Cream Bran Muffins

Serving: 48 mini muffins | Prep: 15mins | Ready in:

Ingredients

- 4 tablespoons butter
- 1/3 cup brown sugar
- 1/4 cup granulated sugar
- 1 whole egg
- 2 egg whites
- 1/3 cup light sour cream
- 1/3 cup nonfat yogurt
- 1/4 cup light molasses
- 1 teaspoon vanilla extract
- 1 cup all-purpose flour
- 1 cup 100% all-bran cereal
- 2 teaspoons baking powder
- 1 teaspoon baking soda
- 2 teaspoons pumpkin pie spice
- 1/4 teaspoon salt
- 1/2 cup raisins
- 2 cups unpeeled apples, coarsely chopped

Direction

- Preheat oven to 400 degrees.
- Line muffin tin with paper cupcake liners.
- Cream butter with both sugars in a large mixing bowl until fluffy.
- Add egg, egg whites, sour cream, yogurt, molasses, and vanilla - mixing until well combined.
- Add flour, bran cereal, baking powder, baking soda, pumpkin pie spice, salt, raisins and apple pieces until just barely combined. Don't overmix - batter will be lumpy.
- Spoon into prepared muffin tin. Bake about 15 minutes if using gem sized muffin cups or 20 minutes if using regular sized muffin cups. Tops of muffins will spring back when lightly touched.

Nutrition Information

- Calories: 49.4
- Sodium: 72.9
- Fiber: 0.6
- Sugar: 5.3
- Protein: 0.9
- Total Fat: 1.4
- Saturated Fat: 0.8
- Total Carbohydrate: 9.1
- Cholesterol: 7

14. Apple And Cinnamon Muffins (Vegan)

Serving: 5 muffins, 5 serving(s) | Prep: 10mins | Ready in:

Ingredients

- Wet mix in a large bowl
- 1 cup unsweetened applesauce
- 1/2 cup raw sugar
- 1 teaspoon vanilla
- Dry Mix
- 1 cup spelt flour
- 2 teaspoons baking powder
- 1/2 teaspoon baking soda
- 1 teaspoon cinnamon
- 1/2 cup walnuts, chopped

Direction

- Combine the wet ingredients. Combine the dry ingredients and sift into the wet mix. Add walnuts. Mix gently but thoroughly.
- Spoon into 5 muffin cases and bake for 20 minutes.

Nutrition Information

- Calories: 179.1
- Sodium: 272.6
- Protein: 1.9
- Fiber: 1.6
- Sugar: 25
- Total Carbohydrate: 28.1
- Cholesterol: 0
- Total Fat: 7.7
- Saturated Fat: 0.7

15. Apple Cheddar Scones

Serving: 10 scones | Prep: 15mins | Ready in:

Ingredients

- 1 cup plain flour
- 1 cup white whole wheat flour
- 3 tablespoons sugar
- 1 1/2 teaspoons baking powder
- 1/2 teaspoon salt
- 1/2 teaspoon ground cinnamon
- 1/4 teaspoon baking soda
- 1 granny smith apple, diced
- 1/2 cup shredded reduced-fat sharp cheddar cheese
- 1/3 cup unsweetened applesauce
- 1 egg
- 1/4 cup skim milk
- 3 tablespoons melted butter

Direction

- Preheat oven to 425 degrees. Line baking sheet with parchment paper.
- Combine flours, sugar, baking powder, salt cinnamon and baking soda. Stir in apple and cheese.
- Whisk applesauce, egg, milk and butter in another bowl. Stir into flour mixture just until moistened.
- Knead dough on floured surface five times. Pat and stretch into an 8 inch circle. Slice into 10 pie-shaped pieces. Place pieces on baking sheet and spray tops with cooking spray. Bake 15 min or until lightly browned.

Nutrition Information

- Calories: 164.5
- Saturated Fat: 2.7
- Sugar: 6.6
- Total Carbohydrate: 26.1
- Fiber: 2.2
- Cholesterol: 29.1
- Protein: 5.2
- Total Fat: 4.8
- Sodium: 278.8

16. Apricot Oat Bran Muffins Low Fat

Serving: 6 Muffins, 6 serving(s) | Prep: 10mins | Ready in:

Ingredients

- 2 cups oat bran
- 1/4 cup packed brown sugar
- 1 tablespoon baking powder
- 2 egg whites
- 1 cup buttermilk
- 1/3 cup molasses
- 1 large apple, peeled, cored and grated
- 3/4 cup finely chopped dried apricot

Direction

- Preheat oven to 400.

- Spray 6 large 3" muffin cups with no-stick spray.
- In large bowl, stir oat bran, brown sugar and baking powder. Make a well in the center.
- In a small bowl, beat the egg whites until foamy. Stir in buttermilk and molasses.
- Add buttermilk mixture to the oat-bran mixture and stir just until moistened. Fold in apples and apricots.
- Spoon the batter into the prepared cups, filling each 3/4 full.
- Bake for 18 to 20 minutes.
- Cool in muffin cups for 5 minutes, then remove and cool on a wire rack.
- NOTE:
- To make standard sized muffins spray 12 2 1/2" muffin cups with no-stick spray, spoon batter into cups. Bake for 15 to 17 minutes.

Nutrition Information

- Calories: 246.6
- Total Fat: 2.7
- Sodium: 256.4
- Protein: 8.6
- Saturated Fat: 0.7
- Fiber: 6.9
- Sugar: 34
- Total Carbohydrate: 61.3
- Cholesterol: 1.6

17. Arabic Honey Glazed Pistachio Muffins

Serving: 5 serving(s) | Prep: 12mins | Ready in:

Ingredients

- 8 1/2 tablespoons all-purpose flour
- 4 tablespoons sugar
- 1/2 teaspoon baking powder
- 1/8 teaspoon baking soda
- 1 pinch salt
- 1 teaspoon ground cardamom
- 3 tablespoons buttermilk
- 1 beaten egg
- 1/2 teaspoon vanilla extract
- 3 tablespoons yogurt
- 3 tablespoons crushed pistachio nuts
- honey, for glaze

Direction

- Pre-heat oven to 350f.
- In a mixing bowl add flour, sugar, baking powder, soda, salt and cardamom and mix well.
- Add buttermilk, egg, vanilla, yogurt and mix well. Fold in pistachios.
- Place 5 liners into a muffin pan and fill 3/4 full with batter. Bake 15-20 mins until lightly browned and toothpick comes out clean.
- Brush tops with honey.

Nutrition Information

- Calories: 136.8
- Saturated Fat: 0.8
- Total Carbohydrate: 22.4
- Cholesterol: 38.7
- Total Fat: 3.5
- Sodium: 127
- Fiber: 0.9
- Sugar: 11.4
- Protein: 4.1

18. Arctic Garden's Blueberry Muffins

Serving: 12 muffins | Prep: 5mins | Ready in:

Ingredients

- 1 3/4 cups whole wheat flour
- 1 tablespoon baking powder
- 1 cup oats
- 1/4 cup brown sugar

- 1 (300 g) packagearctic garden's frozen blueberries (or any other frozen blueberries)
- 1 egg, beaten
- 1 cup unsweetened applesauce
- 1/4 cup orange juice
- 1/4 cup vegetable oil
- 3/4 cup maple syrup

Direction

- Preheat oven 210 C (400 F), and grease muffin pan.
- Combine flour, baking powder, oats, brown sugar, and blueberries.
- In a small bowl combine egg, applesauce, orange juice, vegetable oil and maple syrup.
- Pour all at once the wet ingredients into the dry ingredients, stirring just until moistened.
- Fill the greased muffin pans until 2/3 full, and bake for 25 minutes. Let cool for 2 minutes before removing.

Nutrition Information

- Calories: 257.9
- Total Fat: 6.3
- Sodium: 102
- Fiber: 4.3
- Sugar: 21.9
- Saturated Fat: 0.9
- Total Carbohydrate: 47.9
- Cholesterol: 17.6
- Protein: 5.3

19. Asiago Scones

Serving: 8 scones | Prep: 10mins | Ready in:

Ingredients

- 2 1/2 cups biscuit mix
- 3/4 cup milk
- 2 teaspoons black pepper
- 1 teaspoon salt
- 1 cup shredded asiago cheese
- 1 teaspoon nutmeg
- 1 egg beaten with 1 tsp water
- 1 teaspoon sugar

Direction

- Preheat oven to 350°F.
- Combine all ingredients except for egg and sugar in large bowl.
- Stir until moistened, mixture will be thick.
- Pile mixture into eight small mounds onto a non-stick cookie sheet.
- Brush scones with egg wash and sprinkle with sugar.
- Bake for 12-15 minutes until light golden brown.

Nutrition Information

- Calories: 180.1
- Fiber: 1
- Sugar: 5
- Protein: 3.8
- Total Fat: 6.7
- Saturated Fat: 2.1
- Sodium: 780.7
- Total Carbohydrate: 25.8
- Cholesterol: 4

20. Atlantic City Sour Cream Biscuits

Serving: 12 biscuits, 12 serving(s) | Prep: 10mins | Ready in:

Ingredients

- 2 cups all-purpose flour
- 1 teaspoon baking soda
- 1 teaspoon baking powder
- 1/2 teaspoon salt
- 1 cup fat free sour cream

Direction

- In a medium-large bowl, blend flour, baking soda, baking powder and salt together with a whisk. Add sour cream and mix into a stiff dough.
- Using floured hands, turn dough out onto a floured board. Flour a rolling pin and roll dough to a 1/2-inch thickness. Cut biscuits with a biscuit cutter or simply with the rim of a drinking glass.
- Place biscuits on an ungreased cookie sheet and bake in a pre-heated 400 degree F oven for 15-20 minutes, or until biscuits are golden brown.

Nutrition Information

- Calories: 95.4
- Sodium: 247.8
- Fiber: 0.6
- Total Carbohydrate: 19.2
- Cholesterol: 1.9
- Total Fat: 0.5
- Saturated Fat: 0.2
- Sugar: 1.6
- Protein: 3.2

21. Baker's Chocolatey Banana Muffins

Serving: 24 serving(s) | Prep: 10mins | Ready in:

Ingredients

- 2/3 cup vegetable oil
- 1 cup sugar
- 2 large eggs
- 2 cups mashed bananas
- 2 cups BAKER'S Semi-Sweet Chocolate
- 1 teaspoon salt
- 1 teaspoon cinnamon
- 2 cups flour
- 2 teaspoons baking soda
- 1 cup chopped nuts (, can be added to the batter)

Direction

- Preheat oven to 350.
- In a mixing bowl, whisk together oil, sugar and eggs; stir in bananas and chocolate chips.
- Combine flour, soda, salt and cinnamon; stir into mixture just to moisten.
- Spoon into 24 greased muffin cups.
- Bake 15- 20 minutes.

Nutrition Information

- Calories: 242.4
- Sodium: 247.7
- Sugar: 17.8
- Protein: 3.3
- Total Fat: 13.8
- Saturated Fat: 3.8
- Fiber: 2
- Total Carbohydrate: 29.5
- Cholesterol: 17.6

22. Baking Powder Biscuit

Serving: 6-8 biscuits, 6-8 serving(s) | Prep: 10mins | Ready in:

Ingredients

- 2 cups flour
- 4 teaspoons baking powder
- 1 teaspoon salt
- 2 tablespoons shortening
- 3/4 cup milk

Direction

- Mix dry ingredients and sift twice.
- Work in the shortening with a pastry blender or two knives.
- Add the liquid gradually, mixing to a soft dough.

- You may need to add an extra tablespoon of milk if too dry.
- Toss on floured board, pat to one-half inch in thickness.
- Cut out with a glass or biscuit cutter.
- Bake at 450 degrees for 12-15 minutes.

Nutrition Information

- Calories: 210.5
- Sodium: 645.4
- Sugar: 0.1
- Protein: 5.3
- Total Fat: 5.8
- Saturated Fat: 1.8
- Fiber: 1.1
- Total Carbohydrate: 34
- Cholesterol: 4.3

23. Baking Powder Biscuits

Serving: 4-6 serving(s) | Prep: 10mins | Ready in:

Ingredients

- 2 cups sifted pastry flour
- 1 teaspoon salt
- 4 teaspoons baking powder
- 1 tablespoon chilled shortening or 1 tablespoon butter
- 3/4 cup milk

Direction

- Into 2 cups of sifted pastry flour, sift and mix one level teaspoon of salt and four level teaspoons baking powder.
- Chop in one level tablespoon chilled shortening or butter, wet to a stiff dough with about three-fourths cup milk or half water and half milk.
- Toss out on a floured board, pat it down and roll one-half inch thick. Cut into small rounds and bake in a hot oven (450° F).

Nutrition Information

- Calories: 307.9
- Total Carbohydrate: 56.7
- Protein: 7.1
- Saturated Fat: 1.9
- Sodium: 968.2
- Fiber: 1.2
- Sugar: 0.2
- Total Fat: 5.5
- Cholesterol: 6.4

24. Banana Biscuits

Serving: 10 biscuits | Prep: 10mins | Ready in:

Ingredients

- 1 banana
- 1 cup brown sugar
- 6 tablespoons butter
- 1 (12 ounce) package refrigerated biscuits

Direction

- Melt butter and brown sugar over medium-high heat and set aside.
- Slice the banana into 10-20 slices (round).
- Split a biscuit in two, place 1 or 2 banana slices on a biscuit half, top with the other biscuit half, and press edges together to seal. Repeat for remaining biscuits.
- Place into a 9x9 inch baking pan with sides touching.
- Drizzle brown sugar/butter mixture over biscuits.
- Bake at 350 degrees for 10-14 minutes, until lightly browned.
- Cool for about 2 minutes, then serve.

Nutrition Information

- Calories: 275.1

- Total Fat: 12.1
- Sodium: 435.2
- Total Carbohydrate: 40.2
- Cholesterol: 18.7
- Protein: 2.7
- Saturated Fat: 5.7
- Fiber: 0.6
- Sugar: 25.5

- Saturated Fat: 2.5
- Fiber: 3.2
- Cholesterol: 40.3
- Protein: 4.8
- Total Fat: 10.9
- Total Carbohydrate: 30.6
- Sodium: 228.4
- Sugar: 13.7

25. Banana Cinnamon Walnut Muffins

Serving: 6 muffins | Prep: 30mins | Ready in:

Ingredients

- 1 cup whole wheat flour
- 1/2 teaspoon baking soda
- 1/4 teaspoon salt
- 1 egg
- 3/4 cup ripe banana, mashed
- 1/3 cup sugar
- 2 tablespoons salad oil
- 1/4 cup walnuts, chopped
- 1 tablespoon butter

Direction

- Blend egg, bananas, sugar, and oil.
- Combine dry ingredients separately and add to wet mixture.
- Stir until moistened.
- Let sit in bowl for several minutes for a fluffier muffin.
- Divide between six large muffin cups. Sprinkle walnut bits on muffin tops.
- Bake at 400 for 19 minutes.
- Remove from oven and smear butter on muffin tops (let butter melt with heat of muffins). Enjoy!

Nutrition Information

- Calories: 228.3

26. Banana Miracle Whip Muffins

Serving: 12 serving(s) | Prep: 5mins | Ready in:

Ingredients

- 1/2 cup mashed banana
- 1/2 cup sugar
- 1/2 cup Miracle Whip
- 1 teaspoon vanilla
- 1 cup flour
- 1 teaspoon baking soda
- 1/4 teaspoon salt

Direction

- Mix bananas, sugar, Miracle Whip and vanilla.
- Combine remaining ingredients and blend with banana mixture.
- Bake at 375F for 12-15 minutes.

Nutrition Information

- Calories: 104.2
- Total Carbohydrate: 20
- Cholesterol: 2.8
- Protein: 1.2
- Total Fat: 2.1
- Fiber: 0.5
- Saturated Fat: 0.3
- Sodium: 241.3
- Sugar: 10.6

27. Banana Muffins With Chocolate And Ginger

Serving: 12 large muffins | Prep: 10mins | Ready in:

Ingredients

- 4 medium mashed ripe bananas
- 2 tablespoons vegetable oil
- 1/4 cup plain yogurt
- 1/3 cup brown sugar, packed
- 1 teaspoon salt
- 1 egg
- 1 teaspoon vanilla
- 1 1/2 cups all-purpose flour
- 1 teaspoon baking soda
- 1 teaspoon baking powder
- 1/4 cup crystallized ginger, chopped fine
- 1/2 cup dark chocolate, chopped into small chunks

Direction

- Sift flour with baking soda, powder and salt. Set aside.
- Mash bananas in a large mixing bowl. Add oil, yogurt, egg, and vanilla. Mix. Add brown sugar and blend well.
- Stir in dry ingredients until well mixed but don't over-beat. Add chocolate and crystallized ginger. Spoon into oiled muffin tins.
- Bake at 350' for 15-20 minutes or until muffins spring back when touched in the centre.

Nutrition Information

- Calories: 172.9
- Fiber: 2.4
- Protein: 3.5
- Total Fat: 6
- Saturated Fat: 2.4
- Sodium: 341
- Sugar: 11.1
- Total Carbohydrate: 28.9
- Cholesterol: 16.2

28. Banana Nut Chocolate Chip Scones

Serving: 12 scones | Prep: 10mins | Ready in:

Ingredients

- 3 cups all-purpose flour
- 1/2 cup packed brown sugar
- 2 teaspoons baking powder
- 1/2 teaspoon salt
- 1/4 teaspoon baking soda
- 3 tablespoons butter, cold
- 1/4 cup buttermilk
- 1 teaspoon vanilla extract
- 2 egg whites
- 1 cup banana, mashed
- 1/2 cup chocolate chips
- vegetable oil cooking spray
- 1/3 cup walnuts, coarsely chopped
- 1 tablespoon brown sugar

Direction

- Heat oven to 400.
- In large mixing bowl, combine flour, sugar, baking powder, baking soda salt.
- Cut in butter with a pastry blender until mixture resembles coarse meal set aside. In medium bowl, mix buttermilk, vanilla extract, egg whites the banana.
- Add to dry mixture just until combined, blend in the chocolate chips.
- Place dough on lightly floured surface knead lightly.
- Spray large cookie sheet with cooking spray.
- Pat dough into a 9-inch circle on the cookie sheet.
- Sprinkle the nuts brown sugar over dough and gently press into dough.
- Cut dough into 12 slices.
- Bake 20 minutes.

Nutrition Information

- Calories: 250.3
- Sodium: 224.2
- Fiber: 1.8
- Sugar: 15.8
- Total Fat: 7.5
- Saturated Fat: 3.4
- Total Carbohydrate: 42.1
- Cholesterol: 7.8
- Protein: 5

29. Banana Oat Bran Muffins

Serving: 12 muffins, 12 serving(s) | Prep: 10mins | Ready in:

Ingredients

- 3/4 cup whole wheat pastry flour
- 1/2 cup whole wheat flour
- 1 cup oat bran
- 1/4 cup sugar
- 1/4 cup maple syrup
- 1 tablespoon baking powder
- 1/2 teaspoon salt
- 3/4 cup nonfat yogurt
- 1/4 cup unsweetened applesauce
- 2 egg whites
- 1 teaspoon vanilla
- 3 small ripe bananas, mashed
- 1 cup raisins
- 1/4 cup chopped pecans

Direction

- Preheat oven to 400.
- Combine flour, oat bran, sugar, baking powder and salt in a large bowl.
- Whisk together yogurt, maple syrup, egg whites, vanilla and banana.
- Stir wet mixture into dry mixture just until combined.
- Stir in raisins.
- Divide batter among 12 muffin cups and sprinkle 1 teaspoon of pecans on each.
- Bake until toothpick inserted in centre comes out clean, about 18-20 minutes.
- Transfer to rack to cool.

Nutrition Information

- Calories: 184.8
- Total Fat: 2.6
- Saturated Fat: 0.3
- Fiber: 4.1
- Cholesterol: 0.3
- Protein: 5.4
- Sodium: 211.8
- Sugar: 19.9
- Total Carbohydrate: 40.7

30. Banana Raisin Muffins

Serving: 6 serving(s) | Prep: 10mins | Ready in:

Ingredients

- 1/4 cup sugar
- 1 teaspoon baking soda
- 1/4 teaspoon salt
- 1 1/2 cups whole wheat flour
- 1/4 cup olive oil
- 1/4 cup 1% low-fat milk
- 2 medium bananas, mashed (around 1 cup)
- 1 teaspoon vanilla
- 1/3 cup raisins

Direction

- Preheat oven to 375° degrees.
- In a large bowl add sugar, baking soda, salt, and flour. Stir well to combine dry ingredients.
- Add oil, milk, mashed bananas and vanilla, mix just until flour is moistened. Fold in raisins.

- Using a non-stick muffin pan or muffin papers, fill muffin cups approximately 2/3 full with batter.
- Bake for approximately 15-20 minutes or until golden brown. Remove from pan and let cool.

Nutrition Information

- Calories: 278.9
- Total Fat: 9.8
- Fiber: 5
- Sugar: 18.6
- Total Carbohydrate: 46
- Cholesterol: 0.5
- Saturated Fat: 1.4
- Sodium: 314.1
- Protein: 5.1

31. Banana Zucchini Chocolate Chip Muffins

Serving: 48 muffins | Prep: 0S | Ready in:

Ingredients

- 1/2 cup margarine
- 222 g unsweetened applesauce
- 2 cups white sugar
- 5 eggs
- 4 mashed bananas
- 2 1/4 cups zucchini, grated
- 1 teaspoon vanilla
- 2 teaspoons baking soda
- 2 teaspoons baking powder
- 1/2 teaspoon salt
- 1 tablespoon cinnamon
- 2 3/4 cups whole wheat flour
- 2 cups white flour
- 1 1/2 cups chocolate chips (optional)

Direction

- Cream first 4 ingredient.
- Add bananas, zucchini and vanilla to mixture.
- Mix in baking soda, baking powder, salt and cinnamon.
- Mix in flours and chocolate chips. Mix until all flour is blended.
- If making muffins, line muffin tins with paper and spray with no stick cooking spray.
- For muffins bake at 325 for 18 minutes; for loaf, bake at 350 for 50 minute.

Nutrition Information

- Calories: 111.5
- Saturated Fat: 0.5
- Fiber: 1.4
- Sugar: 9.7
- Total Carbohydrate: 20.5
- Total Fat: 2.6
- Sodium: 122.5
- Cholesterol: 22
- Protein: 2.4

32. Banana Oat Bran Muffins

Serving: 12 muffins | Prep: 10mins | Ready in:

Ingredients

- 1 1/4 cups flour
- 1 cup oat bran
- 1/2 cup sugar
- 1 tablespoon baking powder
- 1/2 teaspoon baking soda
- 1/2 teaspoon salt
- 3/4 cup skim milk
- 1/4 cup unsweetened applesauce
- 1 teaspoon vanilla
- 2 very ripe bananas, chopped

Direction

- Preheat oven to 400 degrees F.
- Combine dry ingredients in large bowl.
- Whisk milk, applesauce and vanilla in medium bowl.

- Add milk mixture to dry ingredients, stirring just until combined.
- Mix in bananas.
- Divide batter among 12 muffin cups (spray muffin pan with nonstick spray first).
- Bake until toothpick inserted in center of muffins comes out clean, about 20 minutes.
- Transfer to a rack to cool.
- Serve warm or at room temperature.

Nutrition Information

- Calories: 126.5
- Sodium: 250.2
- Fiber: 2.1
- Total Carbohydrate: 29.7
- Protein: 3.5
- Total Fat: 0.8
- Sugar: 11.4
- Cholesterol: 0.3
- Saturated Fat: 0.2

33. Banana Praline Muffins

Serving: 12 muffins, 12 serving(s) | Prep: 10mins | Ready in:

Ingredients

- 1/3 cup chopped pecans, toasted
- 3 tablespoons brown sugar
- 1 tablespoon light sour cream
- 3 small ripe bananas
- 1 large egg
- 1 1/2 cups pancake mix
- 1/2 cup sugar
- 2 tablespoons vegetable oil
- cooking spray

Direction

- Stir together pecans, brown sugar and sour cream. Set aside.
- Mash bananas in a medium bowl, add egg and next 3 ingredients, stirring just until dry ingredients are moistened.
- Place paper baking cups in muffin pans and coat cups with cooking spray.
- Spoon batter into muffin cup, filling three fourths full. Carefully spoon pecan mixture evenly in center of each muffin.
- Bake at 400F for 18-20 minutes or until golden. Remove from pans immediately and cool on wire racks.
- Note: You can freeze muffins, if desired. To reheat, microwave at HIGH 1 minute.

Nutrition Information

- Calories: 177.5
- Protein: 2.8
- Total Fat: 5.9
- Sugar: 14.9
- Total Carbohydrate: 29.6
- Cholesterol: 21.5
- Saturated Fat: 0.9
- Sodium: 205.7
- Fiber: 1.4

34. Bananaluscious Muffins

Serving: 21 Muffings, 21 serving(s) | Prep: 10mins | Ready in:

Ingredients

- 3 medium bananas, very ripe mashed
- 1 cup nonfat yogurt
- 1/2 cup brown sugar, lightly packed
- 1/4 cup vegetable oil
- 1 2/3 cups flour
- 2 teaspoons baking soda
- 2 tablespoons ground flax seed meal

Direction

- Preheat oven to 400 degrees F. Prepare a cupcake pan with paper cups or non-stick cooking spray.
- Combine the mashed bananas, yogurt (or sour cream) brown sugar and vegetable oil.
- In another bowl, combine the flour and baking soda. (If using flaxseed, you can toss it in here.).
- Add the wet to the dry ingredients and mix until combined.
- Bake 15-17 minutes. If mini muffins, check at 15 minutes.

Nutrition Information

- Calories: 104.1
- Fiber: 0.9
- Protein: 2
- Sodium: 130.9
- Sugar: 8.1
- Total Carbohydrate: 17.6
- Cholesterol: 0.2
- Total Fat: 3
- Saturated Fat: 0.4

35. Basic Biscuit

Serving: 8 serving(s) | Prep: 10mins | Ready in:

Ingredients

- 2 cups self-rising flour
- 1 -2 tablespoon shortening or 1 -2 tablespoon lard
- 1 cup buttermilk
- 1/2 teaspoon salt (optional)

Direction

- Work the shortening into the flour until it's like coarse crumbs.
- Add the buttermilk and stir until makes a ball in the bowl.
- You can either pinch off the dough or cut it with a biscuit cutter.
- Grease or spray pan.
- Bake in preheated 400 degree oven for 15 to 20 minutes until brown on top.

Nutrition Information

- Calories: 137
- Saturated Fat: 0.6
- Sugar: 1.5
- Cholesterol: 1.2
- Protein: 4.1
- Total Fat: 2.2
- Sodium: 429
- Fiber: 0.8
- Total Carbohydrate: 24.7

36. Basic Carrot Muffins

Serving: 12 muffins, 12 serving(s) | Prep: 5mins | Ready in:

Ingredients

- 1 cup all-purpose flour
- 1 cup whole wheat flour
- 2/3 cup brown sugar, packed
- 1 teaspoon baking powder
- 1/2 teaspoon baking soda
- 1/2 teaspoon salt
- 1/2 teaspoon cinnamon
- 1/4 teaspoon nutmeg
- 2 large eggs, beaten
- 3/4 cup buttermilk or 3/4 cup soured milk
- 1/3 cup cooking oil
- 1 1/2 cups carrots, grated
- white sugar

Direction

- Preheat oven to 375°C.
- Measure first 7 ingredients into a large bowl. Stir and make a well in the center.

- Combine next 4 ingredients in a medium bowl. Mix well. Add to well.
- Add grated carrot. Stir until just moistened.
- Divide evenly among 12 greased muffin cups.
- Top each muffin with some white sugar or some streusel topping. Here is where you can get really creative. Nuts might be nice for some people. Others might want some oatmeal sprinkled on top. You could do many different toppings in one pan.
- Bake for 20 - 22 minutes or until pick comes out clean.
- Let stand in pan for 5 minutes before removing to wire rack to cool.
- **There are a few variations listed in the book.
- Date Nut Carrot Muffins: Stir in 1/2 cup chopped dates and 1/2 cup chopped pecans into buttermilk mixture. The baking time may need to be longer (20-25 minutes total).
- Ginger Oat Carrot Muffins: Reduce Whole wheat flour to 1/2 cup. Add 1/2 cup quick cooking oats. Add 2 tsp finely chopped, peeled gingerroot. Sprinkle tops of muffins with 1/4 cup quick cooking oats before baking. Baking time may need to be longer (20-25 minutes total).

Nutrition Information

- Calories: 196.1
- Sugar: 13.3
- Total Carbohydrate: 29.4
- Cholesterol: 35.9
- Total Fat: 7.4
- Sodium: 222.3
- Protein: 4.1
- Saturated Fat: 1.2
- Fiber: 1.9

37. Basic Cornbread

Serving: 1 8inch square pan, 4-6 serving(s) | Prep: 10mins | Ready in:

Ingredients

- 1 cup cornmeal
- 1 cup flour
- 2 teaspoons baking powder
- 1/2 teaspoon baking soda
- 1 cup yogurt or 1 cup buttermilk
- 1 egg
- 3 tablespoons honey or 3 tablespoons sugar
- 3 tablespoons oil

Direction

- Preheat the oven to 350 degrees F.
- Grease an 8 inch square pan with oil.
- Combine the dry ingredients in a medium sized bowl.
- Combine the wet ingredients [including the sugar or honey] separately.
- Stir the wet mixture into the dry just enough to thoroughly combine.
- Spread into the greased tin.
- Bake for 20 minutes or until the centre is firm to the touch.

Nutrition Information

- Calories: 419.1
- Sodium: 396.5
- Total Carbohydrate: 63.8
- Cholesterol: 60.8
- Protein: 9.4
- Total Fat: 14.8
- Saturated Fat: 3.4
- Fiber: 3.1
- Sugar: 16.2

38. Basic Navajo Fry Bread

Serving: 8 serving(s) | Prep: 10mins | Ready in:

Ingredients

- 3 cups flour

- 1 teaspoon salt
- 1 tablespoon baking powder
- 1 1/2 cups water
- 1 tablespoon shortening
- oil (for frying)

Direction

- Combine dry ingredients in a bowl.
- Cut in the shortening until it resembles crumbs.
- Slowly add water and mix thoroughly until you have a good dough.
- Knead the dough for a few minutes.
- Use flour when needed and break off pieces about the size of a golf ball.
- You flatten these balls to about pancake size and fry in hot oil.
- I don't remember the reason why but the Indians poke a hole in the center of the dough before frying.
- When they are golden, drain on paper towels.

Nutrition Information

- Calories: 185.7
- Sugar: 0.1
- Saturated Fat: 0.5
- Sodium: 428.7
- Fiber: 1.3
- Total Carbohydrate: 36.2
- Cholesterol: 0
- Protein: 4.8
- Total Fat: 2.1

39. Beef And Cheese Biscuit With A Kick

Serving: 6 Biscuits | Prep: 10mins | Ready in:

Ingredients

- 1 cup biscuit batter (your favorite)
- 1/2 cup ground beef, cooked
- 1/2 cup monterey jack pepper cheese (or your favorite)
- 1 jalapeno, chopped (or more)
- cilantro (to garnish)

Direction

- Toss ground beef with minced jalapeños.
- Drop biscuit batter in the bottom of buttered muffin tins or just use silicone muffin tin and skip the buttering.
- Top with ground beef mixture. Add a big pinch of cheese.
- Bake in a 350° oven until the dough is done and the cheese melts, about 15 minutes.
- Sprinkle with chopped cilantro.

Nutrition Information

- Calories: 75.2
- Sugar: 0.1
- Total Carbohydrate: 0.2
- Protein: 5.7
- Fiber: 0.1
- Saturated Fat: 2.9
- Sodium: 62.6
- Cholesterol: 20.8
- Total Fat: 5.6

40. Best Banana Bran Muffins

Serving: 12 large muffins, 12 serving(s) | Prep: 10mins | Ready in:

Ingredients

- 2 large ripe bananas (or 3 med. size)
- 1/2 cup vegetable oil
- 1 cup brown sugar (or 1/2 c. of 'Splenda' brown sugar)
- 1 1/4 cups plain yogurt
- 1 teaspoon baking soda
- 2 eggs
- 1 cup flour

- 2 cups natural bran, powdery stuff. you can also buy just the right amt. at the bulk store (Quaker green box)
- 1/2 cup light raisins or 1/2 cup craisins
- 1/4 cup sunflower seeds

Direction

- Add the baking soda to the yogurt in a larger cup or bowl. Set this aside.
- Beat eggs, oil, mashed bananas and sugar.
- Combine the flour, bran, raisons and sunflower seeds. Add the yogurt/soda mixture to the egg, bananas, then add the flour. Put into paper-lined large muffin tins and bake at 400 degrees for 18 to 20 minutes.

Nutrition Information

- Calories: 291
- Total Fat: 12.9
- Sodium: 160.7
- Fiber: 4.3
- Total Carbohydrate: 43.5
- Cholesterol: 38.6
- Saturated Fat: 2.2
- Sugar: 25.8
- Protein: 5.4

41. Best Cheese Cornbread

Serving: 4 serving(s) | Prep: 5mins | Ready in:

Ingredients

- 1 (14 3/4 ounce) can creamed corn
- 1 (8 1/2 ounce) box Jiffy cornbread mix
- 2/3 cup plain yogurt (can sub buttermilk)
- 1/3 cup aunt jemima pancake mix
- 1 1/2 cups grated cheese (I use mixed cheese)

Direction

- Turn on sandwich maker, waffle iron, iron skillet or greased pan to medium heat.
- Mix all ingredients in a large bowl. Mixture should be thick. I add the cheese last and don't mix it in evenly. I like there to be spots with chunks of melted cheese.
- Scoop the amount you need depending on how you are cooking it. They will fluff up, so don't over fill sandwich maker or waffle iron. Usually about 1-3 minutes on each side. Longer if you like it toasty.
- Serve hot. Enjoy!

Nutrition Information

- Calories: 539.3
- Saturated Fat: 9.4
- Sugar: 5.6
- Protein: 17
- Total Fat: 20.1
- Sodium: 1551.8
- Fiber: 5.6
- Total Carbohydrate: 75.5
- Cholesterol: 35.9

42. Best Ever Banana Muffins

Serving: 12 muffins | Prep: 10mins | Ready in:

Ingredients

- 1 1/2 cups flour, all purpose
- 1 teaspoon baking powder
- 1 teaspoon baking soda
- 1/2 teaspoon salt
- 1 egg
- 3/4 cup sugar
- 1/3 cup butter, melted
- 1 1/2 cups bananas, mashed (3 or 4)

Direction

- Preheat oven to 375F.
- Combine flour, baking powder, baking soda and salt in bowl.

- Beat together egg, sugar, butter, and mashed bananas in another bowl.
- Add to dry ingredients and stir until just moistened.
- Fill greased muffin cups three quarters full.

Nutrition Information

- Calories: 173.3
- Protein: 2.4
- Sodium: 283.6
- Sugar: 14.8
- Total Carbohydrate: 28.8
- Cholesterol: 29
- Total Fat: 5.7
- Saturated Fat: 3.4
- Fiber: 0.9

43. Best Ever Eggless Banana Oatmeal Muffins

Serving: 6 muffins | Prep: 10mins | Ready in:

Ingredients

- 3/4 cup all-purpose flour
- 1/2 cup rolled oats
- 1/4 cup brown sugar, unpacked
- 1 teaspoon baking powder
- 1/2 teaspoon baking soda
- 1/4 teaspoon salt
- 3/8 cup skim milk or 3/8 cup soymilk
- 1/4 cup applesauce
- 1/4 teaspoon vanilla extract
- 1/2 cup mashed banana

Direction

- Preheat oven to 400 degrees F (205 degrees C).
- In a bowl, combine flour, oats, sugar, baking powder, soda, and salt.
- In another large bowl, mix together milk, applesauce, and vanilla.

- Add the mashed bananas, and combine thoroughly.
- Stir the flour mixture into the banana mixture until just combined.
- Lightly grease and dust 6 muffin cups (or line with paper bake cups), and divide the batter among them.
- Bake at 400 degrees F (205 degrees C) for 20 minutes.

Nutrition Information

- Calories: 141.2
- Sugar: 10.6
- Total Carbohydrate: 30.9
- Cholesterol: 0.3
- Saturated Fat: 0.1
- Sodium: 276.9
- Fiber: 1.5
- Total Fat: 0.7
- Protein: 3.3

44. Best Scones

Serving: 12 scones | Prep: 15mins | Ready in:

Ingredients

- 2 cups self-raising flour
- 1 pinch salt
- 30 g butter, cut into small pieces
- 1/2 cup milk
- 1/2 cup water

Direction

- Preheat oven to 220°C Sift flour and salt. Add butter and rub using your fingertips.
- Combine milk and water. Make a well in the center of the flour. Pour liquid all at once. Mix quickly to a soft dough.
- Knead lightly. Press or roll out to form a round about 2 cm thick.

- Cut using a round cutter and place on a greased oven tray and glaze with milk.
- Bake for 10-12 min or until scones sound hollow when tapped.

Nutrition Information

- Calories: 98.1
- Sodium: 297
- Sugar: 0.1
- Cholesterol: 6.8
- Protein: 2.4
- Total Fat: 2.6
- Saturated Fat: 1.5
- Fiber: 0.6
- Total Carbohydrate: 15.9

45. Better Cheddar Biscuits

Serving: 12 buscuits | Prep: 15mins | Ready in:

Ingredients

- 2 1/2 cups baking mix
- 3/4 cup cold milk
- 4 tablespoons cold butter
- 1/4 teaspoon garlic powder
- 1 -1 1/2 cup shredded cheddar cheese
- TOPPING
- 1/4 teaspoon dried parsley
- 1/8 teaspoon garlic powder
- 2 tablespoons melted butter
- 1 pinch salt

Direction

- Preheat oven to 400 degrees.
- Put baking mix in large bowl and use a large fork or pastry cutter to incorporate cold butter into mix (you want pea size balls of butter throughout the mixture.)
- Add cheddar cheese and 1/4 Tsp garlic powder and mix by hand until combined (Being careful not to mush the butter or cheese too much).
- Drop by 1/4 cup portions on ungreased cookie sheet and bake for 15-17 minutes until light brown.
- Melt 2Tbs butter in the microwave with 1/8 Tsp garlic powder and 1/4 Tsp dried parsley flakes and a pinch of salt and brush onto the cooked biscuits.

Nutrition Information

- Calories: 175.2
- Protein: 2.7
- Total Fat: 10.4
- Saturated Fat: 5
- Total Carbohydrate: 17.7
- Sodium: 341.1
- Fiber: 0.6
- Sugar: 3.1
- Cholesterol: 17.9

46. Betty's Of York Tea Room Fat Rascals Fruit Buns/Scones

Serving: 8-10 Fat Rascals | Prep: 10mins | Ready in:

Ingredients

- 100 g butter, softened
- 250 g plain flour
- 75 g currants
- 50 g mixed citrus peels
- 1 1/2 teaspoons baking powder
- 75 g golden caster sugar
- 150 ml whipping cream or 150 ml sour cream or 150 ml creme fraiche
- 1 egg, beaten
- glace cherries, for decoration
- blanched almond, for decoration (whole)

Direction

- Pre-heat the oven to 220C/425F/Gas 7 and grease or line a baking sheet, or a cookie sheet.
- Rub the butter into the flour until it resembles breadcrumbs.
- Add the remaining dry ingredients and mix well.
- Add the cream and mix to a stiff paste - a firm dough.
- Roll the mixture out on a floured board, to about 1" thickness and stamp out rounds, of about 3" in diameter. (You can also shape the fat rascals by hand; take a piece of dough, about the size of a small egg, and make a small ball - flatten it out slightly into bread roll shapes - like a bread bap shape.)
- Arrange them on the greased baking tray and glaze them generously with the beaten egg.
- Then place 2 whole blanched almonds on top with a halved glace cherry for decoration - pushing them down gently into the dough, so they do not fall off during baking!
- Bake for 15 to 20 minutes, or until they have risen and are golden brown.
- Allow to cool on a wire cooling rack.
- Store them in an airtight tin for up to 4 days.

Nutrition Information

- Calories: 371.4
- Cholesterol: 77.6
- Saturated Fat: 10.8
- Fiber: 2.4
- Sodium: 156.9
- Sugar: 15.8
- Total Carbohydrate: 48.5
- Protein: 5.8
- Total Fat: 17.7

47. Bigfatmomma's Better For You Pumpkin Muffins

Serving: 12-14 muffins | Prep: 10mins | Ready in:

Ingredients

- 1/2 cup butter, room temperature
- 3/4 cup sucanat or 3/4 cup dark brown sugar, firmly packed
- 1/3 cup molasses
- 1 egg, room temperature
- 1 cup canned pumpkin
- 1 3/4 cups whole wheat pastry flour
- 1/4 teaspoon salt
- 1 teaspoon baking soda
- 1 1/2 teaspoons cinnamon
- 1/4 teaspoon clove
- 1 teaspoon nutmeg
- 1/4 raisins

Direction

- Preheat oven to 400 degrees.
- Grease muffin tin, or line with paper liners.
- With an electric mixer, cream butter until soft.
- Add sucanat and molasses, and beat until light and fluffy.
- Add egg and pumpkin, stir until well blended.
- Sift flour, salt, soda, cinnamon, cloves and nutmeg into the butter mixture, and fold in, being careful not to over mix.
- Gently fold in raisins.
- Spoon equal amounts into muffin tin.
- Bake until the tops spring back when lightly touched, about 12-15 minutes.
- Let cool in pan 3 minutes before moving to cooling rack.

Nutrition Information

- Calories: 169.3
- Protein: 3.2
- Saturated Fat: 5.1
- Fiber: 2.9
- Sodium: 267.4
- Sugar: 6
- Total Carbohydrate: 21.7
- Cholesterol: 38
- Total Fat: 8.6

48. Bisquick Cinnamon Raisin Biscuits

Serving: 9 serving(s) | Prep: 10mins | Ready in:

Ingredients

- 2 cups Bisquick
- 1/2 cup milk
- 1/3 cup granulated sugar
- 1/3 cup raisins
- 1 teaspoon cinnamon

Direction

- Preheat oven to 425°F.
- Stir all ingredients until soft dough forms.
- Drop by spoonfuls onto ungreased cookie sheet.
- Sprinkle with additional sugar, if desired.
- Bake 10 to 12 minutes or until golden.

Nutrition Information

- Calories: 168.2
- Saturated Fat: 1.4
- Sodium: 347.6
- Fiber: 0.9
- Sugar: 13.7
- Total Fat: 4.6
- Total Carbohydrate: 29.4
- Cholesterol: 2.4
- Protein: 2.8

49. Black Pepper And Bacon Drop Biscuits

Serving: 12 biscuits, 12 serving(s) | Prep: 15mins | Ready in:

Ingredients

- 6 slices bacon
- 2 cups all-purpose flour
- 2 teaspoons baking powder
- 1/2 teaspoon baking soda
- 1 teaspoon sugar
- 3/4 teaspoon salt
- 1 teaspoon fresh coarse ground black pepper
- 1 cup cold buttermilk
- 8 tablespoons unsalted butter, melted and cooled slightly
- 2 tablespoons melted butter, for brushing tops of biscuits

Direction

- Cut bacon in half lengthwise and then crosswise into 1/4-inch pieces; fry in a skillet over medium heat until crisp, 5-7 minutes. Transfer pieces to a paper towel and cool.
- Adjust oven rack to middle position and heat oven to 475°F. Line a large baking sheet with parchment paper.
- Whisk flour, baking powder, baking soda, sugar, salt and pepper in a large bowl. Stir in bacon pieces.
- In a medium bowl, combine cold buttermilk and 8 tablespoons melted butter, stirring until butter forms small clumps.
- This may look like a mistake, but it's one of the secrets of this recipe. The clumps of butter are similar to small bits of cold butter in biscuits prepared by the traditional method. As the butter melts during baking, the steam helps the biscuits rise and gives them a light and fluffy interior.
- Add buttermilk mixture to dry ingredients and stir until just incorporated and batter pulls away from sides of bowl.
- Using a 1/4-cup dry measure, scoop level amounts of batter and drop onto baking sheet (biscuits should measure about 2 1/4-inches in diameter and 1 1/4-inch high). Space biscuits 1 1/2-inces apart.
- Bake until the tops are golden brown and crisp, 12-14 minutes.
- Remove from oven and brush tops with melted butter. Let cool 5 minutes before serving.

- Bring on the gravy!
- Other variations- Omit the bacon and pepper and add:
- Cheddar Scallion - 1/2 cup grated cheddar cheese and 1/4 cup thinly sliced scallions.
- Parmesan Rosemary - 3/4 cup grated Parmesan cheese and 1/2 teaspoons finely minced rosemary.

Nutrition Information

- Calories: 222.9
- Total Fat: 15.1
- Sodium: 389.3
- Sugar: 1.4
- Cholesterol: 34
- Protein: 4.3
- Saturated Fat: 7.9
- Fiber: 0.6
- Total Carbohydrate: 17.6

50. Blackberry Scones

Serving: 8 serving(s) | Prep: 15mins | Ready in:

Ingredients

- 1/2 cup low-fat milk
- 1 egg
- 2 cups flour
- 2 teaspoons baking powder
- 1/2 teaspoon salt
- 1/4 cup cold butter, cubed
- 3 tablespoons white sugar
- 1 cup frozen blackberrie

Direction

- Preheat oven to 425 degrees Fahrenheit. Whisk the milk and the egg together until frothy and then set aside. In a large bowl, blend the flour, baking powder, and salt. Add the butter and blend the mixture with your hands until you have no lumps larger than a pea. Add the sugar and the blackberries and toss about until the blackberries are coated with the flour mixture. Add the egg mixture slowly until the dough comes together. Leave any remaining egg mixture to brush on as glaze.
- Turn dough out onto a clean counter and knead it no more than 12 times. Pat dough into a round approximately 1/2 an inch thick, and cut into 8 wedges. Place on an ungreased baking sheet or a Silpat. Using a pastry brush, glaze wedges with remaining egg mixture. Bake for 10-15 minutes, or until golden. Cool on a wire rack.

Nutrition Information

- Calories: 210.9
- Total Fat: 6.9
- Cholesterol: 39.3
- Protein: 4.8
- Saturated Fat: 4
- Sodium: 303.2
- Fiber: 1.8
- Sugar: 7.6
- Total Carbohydrate: 32.6

51. Blue Cornbread

Serving: 8 serving(s) | Prep: 10mins | Ready in:

Ingredients

- 1 cup blue cornmeal
- 1/2 cup whole wheat pastry flour
- 1 1/2 teaspoons baking powder
- 1/4 teaspoon salt (optional)
- 1 tablespoon honey or 1 tablespoon maple syrup
- 1 egg, beaten
- 1/3 cup nonfat dry milk powder
- 2/3 cup water
- 1 tablespoon cooking oil

Direction

- Lightly spray an 8- to 9-inch cast iron skillet with cooking spray and drizzle with the 1 tablespoon cooking oil.
- Place the skillet in the oven while it preheats.
- Preheat oven to 425°F.
- In a medium size bowl, combine dry ingredients.
- Combine liquids and slowly add to combined dry ingredients, mixing well.
- Pour into prepared pan and bake at 425°F for 15-20 minutes, until top and sides become golden brown.

Nutrition Information

- Calories: 136.8
- Saturated Fat: 0.6
- Protein: 5.2
- Fiber: 2.2
- Sugar: 5.1
- Total Carbohydrate: 22.2
- Cholesterol: 27.4
- Total Fat: 3.3
- Sodium: 105.5

52. Blueberry Cottage Cheese Muffins

Serving: 10 muffins | Prep: 15mins | Ready in:

Ingredients

- 1/4 cup low fat cottage cheese
- 1 egg
- 3/4 cup all-purpose flour
- 1/2 teaspoon salt
- 1 1/4 teaspoons baking powder
- 2 tablespoons granulated sugar (optional) or 2 tablespoons equivalent sugar substitute (optional)
- 1/3 cup skim milk
- 1 cup fresh blueberries, washed

Direction

- Use a fork to blend the cottage cheese and egg together. Add the flour, salt, baking powder and sugar; stir to combine.
- Add milk and stir lightly, then gently stir in the blueberries.
- Spoon into 10 muffin cups and bake in a preheated 425 degree oven for 15-18 minutes.

Nutrition Information

- Calories: 58.5
- Total Carbohydrate: 10.1
- Cholesterol: 21.8
- Protein: 2.8
- Sodium: 196.8
- Fiber: 0.6
- Total Fat: 0.8
- Saturated Fat: 0.3
- Sugar: 1.5

53. Blueberry Doughnut Muffins

Serving: 24 serving(s) | Prep: 10mins | Ready in:

Ingredients

- 2 1/4 cups flour
- 1 tablespoon baking powder
- 1 teaspoon baking soda
- 1 pinch salt
- 1/4 teaspoon nutmeg
- 4 tablespoons brown sugar
- 1 cup sour cream
- 1 egg
- 1/4 cup melted butter
- 1 teaspoon vanilla
- 1/2 cup frozen blueberries
- Topping
- 1 cup white sugar
- 1/2 tablespoon cinnamon (full)
- 1/2-1 cup melted butter

Direction

- Preheat oven to 400°F and grease 24 mini muffin tins (this recipe works the best with mini muffins, but use large if you prefer, you will have adjust your cooking time accordingly).
- Combine dry ingredients.
- Combine wet ingredients in a separate bowl and stir with a whisk, and then stir blueberries into this.
- Add wet ingredients to dry and blend but do not over mix.
- Spoon muffins into tins, filling almost to top to make a nice crown.
- Bake for about 12-15 minutes.
- Let cool in tins for 2 minutes, and then remove and place on rack to cool an additional 5 minutes.
- Stir sugar and cinnamon together.
- Dip muffins all the way in butter and then roll in sugar mixture. Serve at once.

Nutrition Information

- Calories: 163.2
- Cholesterol: 28.3
- Total Fat: 8.1
- Saturated Fat: 5
- Sodium: 154.4
- Fiber: 0.5
- Sugar: 11.6
- Total Carbohydrate: 21.3
- Protein: 1.9

54. Blueberry English Scones

Serving: 12 serving(s) | Prep: 10mins | Ready in:

Ingredients

- 2 cups all-purpose flour
- 1/4 cup sugar
- 2 1/2 teaspoons baking powder
- 1/2 teaspoon baking soda
- 1/2 teaspoon salt
- 1/4 cup butter
- 3/4 cup fresh blueberries
- 1 cup milk

Direction

- Preheat oven to 425°F Grease a baking tray or line the baking tray with parchment paper.
- Mix the flour, sugar, baking powder, baking soda and salt together. Cut in the butter until the mixture resembles fine breadcrumbs. Stir in the blueberries.
- Add the milk and mix to make a smooth dough (you may not need all of the milk). Knead lightly for ten seconds on a lightly floured surface. Roll to about 3/4" thick and either cut into individual scones or cut into wedges.
- Bake for approximately 8-12 minutes.

Nutrition Information

- Calories: 144.5
- Cholesterol: 13
- Protein: 2.9
- Total Fat: 4.8
- Sodium: 262.7
- Total Carbohydrate: 22.6
- Saturated Fat: 2.9
- Fiber: 0.8
- Sugar: 5.1

55. Blueberry Muffins Low Calorie

Serving: 12 muffins, 12 serving(s) | Prep: 10mins | Ready in:

Ingredients

- 1/2 cup all-purpose flour
- 1/4 cup sugar
- 1 1/2 teaspoons baking powder
- 1/4 teaspoon salt
- 2 egg whites

- 1/3 cup orange juice
- 2 tablespoons applesauce (unflavored)
- 1 teaspoon vanilla
- 1 cup blueberries (fresh or frozen)

Direction

- Mix together flour, sugar, baking powder and salt in a medium-size bowl.
- In a small bowl beat egg whites, orange juice, oil and vanilla
- Add to dry ingredients
- Fold in blueberries.
- Fill muffin cups (sprayed with non-stick cooking spray) about half full.
- Bake at 400 degrees for 17 minutes or until golden brown.

Nutrition Information

- Calories: 51.2
- Total Fat: 0.1
- Saturated Fat: 0
- Sodium: 104
- Fiber: 0.5
- Protein: 1.3
- Sugar: 6
- Total Carbohydrate: 11.3
- Cholesterol: 0

56. Blueberry Oat Bran Muffins

Serving: 12 serving(s) | Prep: 10mins | Ready in:

Ingredients

- 2 cups oat bran
- 1/3 cup Splenda sugar substitute
- 2 teaspoons baking powder
- 1/4 teaspoon baking soda
- 1/2 cup low-fat vanilla yogurt
- 1/2 cup orange juice
- 1/2 cup egg substitute
- 2 tablespoons canola oil or 2 tablespoons walnut oil
- 1 cup fresh blueberries or 1 cup frozen blueberries
- 2 teaspoons cinnamon

Direction

- Mix dry ingredients in large bowl. Add combined wet ingredients. Fold in blueberries. Coat bottoms only of muffin tin. Fill 3/4 full. Bake at 350°F for about 15 minutes.
- Allow to sit for 5 minutes before removing from pan.
- These freeze well.

Nutrition Information

- Calories: 89.5
- Total Fat: 4
- Saturated Fat: 0.5
- Fiber: 2.9
- Sugar: 3.8
- Protein: 4.7
- Sodium: 112.9
- Total Carbohydrate: 15.2
- Cholesterol: 0.6

57. Blueberry And Lemon Muffins

Serving: 12 muffins | Prep: 5mins | Ready in:

Ingredients

- 2 cups self raising flour
- 1/4 cup caster sugar
- 1 cup skim milk
- 1 egg, lightly beaten
- 1 teaspoon vanilla essence
- 2 tablespoons low-fat butter, melted
- 3 teaspoons lemon rind, grated
- 150 g blueberries

Direction

- Preheat oven to 200deg Celsius.
- Coat a 12 hole (1/2 c capacity) muffin tin with cooking spray.
- Sift flour into bowl and add sugar.
- Combine milk, egg, vanilla, melted butter and lemon rind.
- Pour into the flour mixture and stir until just smooth. The mixture will look lumpy but do not over-beat.
- Stir through blueberries (leave a couple for decoration on the top).
- Spoon mixture into muffin tin and bake 18-20mins until golden.
- Let cool for 5mins before turning out onto a wire rack.

Nutrition Information

- Calories: 114.9
- Sodium: 18.5
- Cholesterol: 18
- Saturated Fat: 0.2
- Fiber: 0.9
- Sugar: 5.6
- Total Carbohydrate: 23.2
- Protein: 3.6
- Total Fat: 0.7

58. Bran Muffins Low Cal

Serving: 12 Muffins, 12 serving(s) | Prep: 15mins | Ready in:

Ingredients

- 3 cups natural bran
- 2 cups buttermilk
- 2/3 cup raisins
- 1/2 cup unsweetened applesauce
- 1/2 cup Splenda granular
- 1/4 cup molasses
- 2 eggs, beaten
- 1 1/4 cups whole wheat flour
- 1 teaspoon salt
- 2 teaspoons baking soda

Direction

- In medium bowl stir together bran, buttermilk and raisins, let soak for 10 minutes.
- Spray muffin tins with nonstick cooking spray, preheat oven to 350. In mixing bowl add Splenda, molasses, applesauce, eggs and mix on low speed till well blended. Add buttermilk mixture and mix on medium speed for 1 minute.
- Add flour, baking soda and salt and mix on low speed till incorporated. Increase speed to medium and mix for 3 minutes. Divide mixture into 12 muffin tins, bake for 15 - 20 minutes.

Nutrition Information

- Calories: 158.8
- Fiber: 6.3
- Sugar: 13.1
- Cholesterol: 36.9
- Protein: 6.3
- Total Fat: 2.2
- Saturated Fat: 0.6
- Sodium: 498.7
- Total Carbohydrate: 35

59. Breakfast Oatmeal Protein Muffins

Serving: 4 muffins, 1 serving(s) | Prep: 10mins | Ready in:

Ingredients

- 1/2 cup rolled oats
- 1 teaspoon baking soda
- 1/2 teaspoon pumpkin pie spice
- 1/2 banana, mashed

- 1 pinch salt
- 2 egg whites
- 1 egg

Direction

- Mix together dry ingredients.
- Mash banana.
- Add eggs to banana and beat slightly.
- Add wet ingredients to dry and mix until it is all incorporated.
- Pour into prepared muffin tins or baking cups.
- Bake for 16 minutes at 350 degrees.

Nutrition Information

- Calories: 314.7
- Total Fat: 7.8
- Saturated Fat: 2.1
- Sodium: 1597.6
- Fiber: 5.8
- Sugar: 8.3
- Total Carbohydrate: 42.3
- Cholesterol: 186
- Protein: 19.5

60. Breakfast Potato Muffins #5FIX

Serving: 12 Muffins, 12 serving(s) | Prep: 10mins | Ready in:

Ingredients

- 20 ounces Simply Potatoes® Shredded Hash Browns
- 1/2 cup salted butter, cold
- 1 cup colby-monterey jack cheese, shredded
- 5 eggs
- 1 teaspoon garlic salt

Direction

- Preheat oven to 350 degrees F.
- In a bowl beat the eggs until mixed.
- Mix in cold butter leaving small chunks of it in the mixture.
- Add garlic powder and mix well.
- Add the potatoes. Coat all the potatoes with egg mixture.
- Mix in cheddar cheese.
- Use a muffin pan that makes 12 muffins. Put potato mixture evenly into the 12 muffin holes and pack down slightly.
- Bake for 25 minutes.
- Remove and let cool slightly and serve.
- For a healthier option use light butter, light cheese, and egg whites.

Nutrition Information

- Calories: 133.6
- Saturated Fat: 7.3
- Total Carbohydrate: 0.4
- Total Fat: 12.5
- Sodium: 147.7
- Fiber: 0
- Sugar: 0.1
- Cholesterol: 106.2
- Protein: 5

61. British Yorkshire Pudding

Serving: 6 serving(s) | Prep: 5mins | Ready in:

Ingredients

- 2 eggs
- 1 egg white
- 4 ounces plain flour
- 1/2 pint milk
- 1 pinch salt

Direction

- Put flour into a mixing bowl.
- Crack in eggs.
- Mix in egg white.
- Gradually add milk.

- Pop in pinch of salt.
- Whisk all ingredients together until well mixed, light and fluffy.
- Meanwhile put muffin tin in oven with vegetable oil in the bottom. Heat on the highest oven setting until oil smokes. Add batter mixture and leave in oven for 20 minutes until crisp and brown and well risen. This mixture will fill six large muffin inserts. Warning--do not open oven during cooking or they will sink. Enjoy.

Nutrition Information

- Calories: 126.2
- Total Fat: 3.4
- Saturated Fat: 1.5
- Sodium: 78.6
- Fiber: 0.5
- Cholesterol: 76.2
- Protein: 6.1
- Sugar: 0.2
- Total Carbohydrate: 17.3

62. BunnyLovingCook's Basic Easy Muffin Recipe

Serving: 12 mufins, 12 serving(s) | Prep: 10mins | Ready in:

Ingredients

- 2 cups flour
- 1/2 cup sugar
- 1 tablespoon baking powder
- 1/2 teaspoon salt
- 3/4 cup milk
- 1/3 cup oil
- 1 egg

Direction

- Preheat oven to 400.
- Mix all ingredients.
- Pour into a greased muffin pan.
- Cook for 15 minutes.
- Serve.

Nutrition Information

- Calories: 177.9
- Cholesterol: 17.6
- Total Fat: 7.2
- Saturated Fat: 1.3
- Total Carbohydrate: 25.2
- Sugar: 8.4
- Protein: 3.2
- Sodium: 201.6
- Fiber: 0.6

63. Butterscotch Pudding Muffins

Serving: 12 muffins | Prep: 0S | Ready in:

Ingredients

- nonstick cooking spray or paper baking cup
- 2 cups all-purpose flour
- 2/3 cup sugar
- 1 (3 ounce) package butterscotch pudding mix (not instant)
- 1 tablespoon baking powder
- 1/2 teaspoon salt
- 1 large egg, at room temperature
- 1 cup milk (whole, lowfat or nonfat)
- 4 tablespoons unsalted butter, melted and cooled
- 1 teaspoon vanilla
- 1 cup butterscotch chips

Direction

- Position the rack in the center of the oven and preheat oven to 400°F. To prepare the muffin tins, spray the indentions and the rims around them with nonstick spray or line the indentations with paper muffin cups. If using

silicon muffin tins, spray as directed, then place them on a baking sheet.
- Whisk the flour, sugar, pudding mix, baking powder, and salt in a medium bowl until uniform. Set aside.
- In a large bowl, whisk the egg, milk, melted butter, and vanilla until light and smooth. Stir in the butterscotch chips with a wooden spoon, then quickly stir in the flour mixture until moistened.
- Fill the prepared tins three quarters full. Use additional greased tins or small, oven safe, greased ramekins for any leftover batter, or reserve the batter for a second baking. Bake for 20 minutes, or until muffins are well browned with smooth round tops. A toothpick inserted in the center of one muffin should come out with a few moist crumbs attached.
- Set the pan on a wire rack to cool for 10 minutes. Gently tip each muffin to the side to make sure it isn't stuck. If it is, gently rock it back and forth to release it. Remove the muffins from the pan and cool them for 5 minutes more on the rack before serving. If storing or freezing, cool them completely before sealing in an airtight container or freezer safe plastic bags. The muffins will stay fresh for up to 2 days at room temperature or up to 2 months in the freezer.

Nutrition Information

- Calories: 249.9
- Fiber: 0.6
- Sugar: 20.8
- Total Carbohydrate: 37.8
- Protein: 3.7
- Total Fat: 9.3
- Saturated Fat: 6.5
- Sodium: 217
- Cholesterol: 30.6

64. Butterscotch Biscuits

Serving: 24 biscuits, 24 serving(s) | Prep: 10mins | Ready in:

Ingredients

- 1 cup brown sugar
- 2 1/2 cups self-raising flour
- 1 cup softened butter
- 2 teaspoons vanilla essence
- 2 tablespoons golden syrup

Direction

- Preheat oven to 160 degrees.
- Combine all ingredients.
- Roll into small balls on a greased flat tray
- Using a fork flatten them slightly.

Nutrition Information

- Calories: 154.7
- Sodium: 224.6
- Fiber: 0.3
- Sugar: 9.4
- Cholesterol: 20.3
- Protein: 1.4
- Total Fat: 7.8
- Saturated Fat: 4.9
- Total Carbohydrate: 20

65. Cajun Biscuits

Serving: 6 serving(s) | Prep: 15mins | Ready in:

Ingredients

- 2 1/3 cups bisquick baking mix
- 1 teaspoon mustard
- 3/4 teaspoon cracked pepper
- 1/2 teaspoon cayenne pepper
- 1/2 teaspoon garlic powder
- 2/3 cup milk

- 1 tablespoon butter or 1 tablespoon margarine, melted

Direction

- Preheat oven to 450 degrees.
- Combine baking mix, mustard powder, cracked pepper, cayenne, and garlic powder.
- Stir in milk until combined and dough just forms.
- Turn dough out onto work surface dusted with additional baking mix; roll out to 3/4-inch thickness.
- Using 2-1/2 inch round cutter, cut out 6 biscuits, rerolling scraps.
- Place on ungreased baking sheet.
- Bake 8-10 minutes or until golden.
- Brush tops with melted butter; serve warm with additional butter, if desired.

Nutrition Information

- Calories: 236.5
- Total Fat: 10.2
- Saturated Fat: 3.7
- Fiber: 1.1
- Cholesterol: 9.8
- Protein: 4.8
- Sodium: 631.9
- Sugar: 5.5
- Total Carbohydrate: 31.3

66. Campfire Muffins

Serving: 12 serving(s) | Prep: 10mins | Ready in:

Ingredients

- 6 oranges
- 2 (7 ounce) packages blueberry muffin mix (or any flavor)

Direction

- Cut oranges in half.
- Scoop out the orange segments to eat alone.
- Reserve the hollow peel shells.
- Prepare the muffin mix according to the package directions.
- Fill the orange peel cups half full of batter.
- Wrap each one loosely with heavy duty aluminum foil.
- Place in hot coals, making sure that the batter side stays up.
- Cook 6-10 minutes until muffins are done.
- Adding a few berries to the batter adds excellent flavor.
- Note: Use 3 oranges per package of muffin mix.

Nutrition Information

- Calories: 152.1
- Total Fat: 3.4
- Saturated Fat: 0.8
- Sodium: 181.6
- Sugar: 6.1
- Total Carbohydrate: 28.6
- Cholesterol: 0
- Protein: 2.2
- Fiber: 1.6

67. Cara Cara Orange Glazed Scones

Serving: 24 medium-size, 6 serving(s) | Prep: 10mins | Ready in:

Ingredients

- 3 cups all-purpose flour
- 1 tablespoon baking powder
- 1/4 teaspoon baking soda
- 1/2 teaspoon kosher salt
- 1/4 tablespoon granulated sugar
- 1/4 cup vegetable oil
- 1 cup water
- 1 teaspoon vanilla

Direction

- Pre-heat oven to 400°.
- Whisk dry ingredients together and place in the bowl of a food processor.
- Running on lowest setting, slowly add oil, water and vanilla until combined and dough has formed.
- Lightly flour surface and pour out dough, gently kneading 1-2 minutes.
- Roll dough out to your desired thickness and cut with biscuit cutters.
- Place on parchment lined baking sheet and bake for 12-15 minutes (depending on size) until golden brown.
- Remove from oven and dip or drizzle with orange glaze while warm.
- For orange glaze: whisk 2 cups of powdered sugar with the zest and juice of one small orange (about 3 tablespoons) and a dash of vanilla to your desired consistency.

Nutrition Information

- Calories: 313
- Total Fat: 9.7
- Saturated Fat: 1.3
- Fiber: 1.7
- Cholesterol: 0
- Sodium: 430.3
- Sugar: 0.8
- Total Carbohydrate: 48.9
- Protein: 6.5

68. Caramel Scones By June

Serving: 12 serving(s) | Prep: 10mins | Ready in:

Ingredients

- 2 cups self raising flour
- 1/4 teaspoon salt
- 4 tablespoons powdered milk
- 4 tablespoons sugar
- 4 tablespoons coconut
- 30 g butter
- 3/4 cup water
- 2 tablespoons butter, extra
- 2 tablespoons brown sugar

Direction

- Heat oven to 220°C.
- Melt extra 2 tablespoons of butter and brown sugar together (I use the microwave).
- Mix flour, salt, milk powder, sugar, coconut, butter and water to a soft dough.
- Roll and cut into 12 rounds.
- Press a thumb hole in the top of each round.
- Fill with melted butter mixture.
- Cook for 10-15 minutes or until cooked through.

Nutrition Information

- Calories: 167.1
- Fiber: 1
- Sugar: 7.7
- Total Fat: 6.6
- Saturated Fat: 4.6
- Sodium: 88.9
- Total Carbohydrate: 24
- Cholesterol: 13
- Protein: 3.1

69. Carrot Pineapple Muffins

Serving: 12 large muffins, 12 serving(s) | Prep: 10mins | Ready in:

Ingredients

- 1 cup all-purpose flour
- 1 cup whole wheat flour or 1 cup barley flour
- 3/4 cup brown sugar, packed
- 1 teaspoon baking powder
- 1 teaspoon baking soda
- 1/2 teaspoon salt

- 1 - 1 1/2 teaspoon cinnamon
- 1/2 teaspoon nutmeg (optional)
- 2 eggs
- 1 tablespoon canola oil
- 3/4 cup applesauce
- 0.5 (398 ml) can crushed pineapple in juice
- 1 cup packed grated carrot (approximately 3 carrots)

Direction

- Preheat oven to 400*.
- Grate carrots until you have 1 cup.
- Blend pineapple until smooth (optional).
- Beat eggs in a bowl, then add oil, applesauce and pineapple.
- Measure all dry ingredients into another bowl. Mix thoroughly. Break any chunks of brown sugar with a spoon.
- Add carrots to dry bowl.
- Mix both wet and dry bowls very well.
- Add the dry ingredients to the wet. Not over-mixing this stage is important for fluffy muffins. In about ten big strokes, gently mix the wet and dry.
- Oil muffin tins with cooking spray or butter on paper towel, or use paper liners.
- Fill 12 large muffins or 48 mini muffins to 3/4 full.
- Using paper towel, wipe off batter spilled on the pan. This makes muffins easier to remove later.
- Bake for 15-20 minutes for mini muffins or 25-35 minutes for large ones, until a toothpick or knife inserted in the centre comes out clean and muffin tops are puffy and golden brown.
- Remove muffins from oven, and leave to sit in the pan for 10 minutes before emptying pan by running the handle of a spoon around each muffin and gently lifting.

Nutrition Information

- Calories: 174.1
- Fiber: 2.1
- Total Fat: 2.4
- Sodium: 260.1
- Sugar: 16.5
- Total Carbohydrate: 35.9
- Cholesterol: 31
- Protein: 3.7
- Saturated Fat: 0.4

70. Carrot Raisin Bran Muffins

Serving: 24 muffins, 24 serving(s) | Prep: 10mins | Ready in:

Ingredients

- 4 1/2 cups oat bran
- 2 tablespoons baking powder
- 1 1/2 cups milk
- 1/2 cup egg substitute
- 6 carrots, shredded
- 3/4 cup raisins
- 3/4 cup molasses
- 4 tablespoons canola oil
- optional spices
- ground cinnamon (optional)
- ground cardamom (optional)
- ground cloves (optional)
- ground allspice (optional)

Direction

- Preheat oven to 425°F
- Combine oat bran and baking powder.
- Mix in remaining ingredients.
- Add optional spices to taste, approximately 1/2 to 1 teaspoon each, in any combination.
- Pour mixture into 24 muffin tins (either oiled or lined with paper muffin cups).
- Bake about 15 minutes, or until a toothpick inserted into muffins comes out clean.

Nutrition Information

- Calories: 129.1
- Protein: 4.5

- Total Fat: 4.4
- Saturated Fat: 0.8
- Sodium: 123.1
- Total Carbohydrate: 25.6
- Fiber: 3.3
- Sugar: 9.5
- Cholesterol: 2.2

71. Carrot And Bran Muffins

Serving: 12 muffins, 12 serving(s) | Prep: 10mins | Ready in:

Ingredients

- 1 cup all-bran cereal, crushed
- 3/4 cup whole wheat flour
- 3/4 cup all-purpose flour
- 1/2 teaspoon cinnamon
- 1/2 teaspoon baking soda
- 1 teaspoon baking powder
- 3 tablespoons brown sugar
- 1/4 teaspoon salt
- 2 egg whites, lightly beaten
- 2 tablespoons vegetable oil
- 1/3 cup applesauce
- 1 tablespoon lemon juice
- 1 cup carrot, grated
- 1/2 cup raisins

Direction

- Pre heat oven to 375. Spray twelve cup muffin pan with oil spray. (I use 24 cup mini muffin pan).
- Combine bran flakes with whole-wheat and al-purpose flours, cinnamon, soda, baking powder, sugar and salt.
- In separate bowl, blend egg whites, oil, buttermilk, apple sauce and lemon juice.
- Combine with dry ingredients. Stir in carrots and raisins until combined.
- Spoon into muffin cups.
- Bake 20 minutes until risen and golden.

Nutrition Information

- Calories: 131.9
- Sodium: 165
- Total Carbohydrate: 26.1
- Saturated Fat: 0.4
- Fiber: 3.2
- Sugar: 8.4
- Cholesterol: 0
- Protein: 3.4
- Total Fat: 2.9

72. Carrot And Date Muffins Gluten Free

Serving: 12 muffins | Prep: 10mins | Ready in:

Ingredients

- 2 medium carrots, peeled and coarsely chopped
- 1 cup chopped pitted dates
- 1/2 cup chopped walnuts
- 1/4 cup melted virgin coconut or 1/4 cup high-heat sunflower oil
- 2 eggs, lightly beaten
- 1/4 cup plus 2 tablespoons pure maple syrup
- 1 1/2 cupselfraising gluten-free flour
- 1/2 teaspoon ground cinnamon
- 1/2 teaspoon freshly grated nutmeg
- 1/2 teaspoon sea salt

Direction

- Line 12 muffin cups with paper liners or oil with natural cooking spray and set aside.
- Preheat oven to 375°F
- Place carrots and dates in the bowl of a food processor. Pulse and then blend until finely chopped. Add walnuts and pulse to finely chop.
- Transfer to a bowl; add oil, eggs and maple syrup, stir to combine completely. In a separate bowl, combine all remaining dry ingredients.

- Pour liquid ingredients over dry ingredients and stir until just combined. Spoon batter into prepared muffin tins and bake for 20 to 25 minutes or until a toothpick inserted in the center of a muffin comes out clean.
- Cool on a wire rack.

Nutrition Information

- Calories: 112.1
- Protein: 2.3
- Sodium: 117.6
- Fiber: 2
- Cholesterol: 31
- Total Carbohydrate: 15.8
- Total Fat: 5.2
- Saturated Fat: 1.6
- Sugar: 12.5

73. Carrot And Poppy Seed Muffins

Serving: 8 muffins | Prep: 5mins | Ready in:

Ingredients

- 150 g self raising flour, sifted
- 150 g brown sugar
- 1 teaspoon ground cinnamon
- 2 eggs, lightly beaten
- 1/2 cup canola oil or 1/2 cup vegetable oil
- 2 cups grated carrots (about 2 large carrots)
- 1 1/2 tablespoons poppy seeds

Direction

- Pre heat oven to 180°C.
- Combine all dry ingredients and carrots in bowl.
- In separate bowl mix oil and eggs together, and then add to dry ingredients, mix till combined. (Don't over mix).
- Divide the mixture into muffin tins that have been oiled lightly with cooking spray.
- Bake in oven for 25 minutes or until skewer comes out clean.
- Cool in pan for a few minutes before transferring to wire rack to cook.

Nutrition Information

- Calories: 315.6
- Total Carbohydrate: 39.7
- Cholesterol: 46.5
- Protein: 4.6
- Saturated Fat: 1.5
- Sugar: 19.7
- Sodium: 42.9
- Fiber: 1.9
- Total Fat: 15.8

74. Carver Brewing Company Raspberry Bran Muffins

Serving: 24 muffins, 24 serving(s) | Prep: 15mins | Ready in:

Ingredients

- 2 1/2 cups wheat bran
- 1 cup pastry flour
- 1/2 cup whole wheat flour
- 1/4 cup packed brown sugar
- 2 1/2 teaspoons baking soda
- 1 cup buttermilk
- 1/2 cup canola oil
- 1/4 cup blackstrap molasses
- 1/4 cup honey
- 4 eggs
- 1 1/2 cups frozen raspberries

Direction

- Preheat oven to 400 degrees F.
- Butter and flour muffin tins or line with paper liners.
- In a large mixing bowl, combine wheat bran, pastry flour, whole-wheat flour, brown sugar

and baking soda, tossing with a fork to incorporate air. Set aside.
- In a smaller bowl, whisk together the buttermilk, canola oil, molasses, honey and eggs.
- Stir wet ingredients into dry ingredients until barely blended. Fold in frozen raspberries.
- Fill tins about two-thirds full. Bake for 15 minutes, or until muffins spring back when touched. Cool in tins.

Nutrition Information

- Calories: 142.2
- Total Fat: 5.8
- Sodium: 156.9
- Fiber: 3.7
- Sugar: 9.1
- Cholesterol: 35.7
- Saturated Fat: 0.7
- Total Carbohydrate: 22
- Protein: 3.3

75. Cheddar And Poppy Seed Potato Scones

Serving: 12-16 serving(s) | Prep: 15mins | Ready in:

Ingredients

- 1 1/2 cups whole wheat flour
- 1 1/2 cups white flour
- 1 tablespoon baking powder
- 1 teaspoon salt
- 2 teaspoons sugar
- 1/2 cup butter, cut into chunks
- 1 cup cooked shredded potato
- 1 cup shredded sharp cheddar cheese
- 2 tablespoons poppy seeds
- 2 teaspoons dried dill
- 1/2-3/4 cup cold milk
- melted butter

Direction

- Preheat oven to 425*F.
- Lightly grease a baking sheet.
- In a large mixing bowl, combine the two flours together with baking powder, salt and sugar.
- Using a pastry blender (or your hands), cut butter into flour mixture until crumbly.
- Stir in the shredded potatoes, cheese, poppy seeds and dill.
- Make a well in the center and add enough milk to make a soft dough (adding more milk as needed).
- Turn out onto a lightly floured work surface and gently knead several times.
- Pat into two 6 to 8-inch rounds about 1-inch thick.
- Cut each into 6 to 8 wedges.
- Place on baking sheet.
- Brush with melted butter.
- Bake until lightly golden, about 12-16 minutes.

Nutrition Information

- Calories: 241.2
- Cholesterol: 31.6
- Total Fat: 12.3
- Sodium: 405
- Fiber: 2.7
- Total Carbohydrate: 27
- Protein: 7
- Saturated Fat: 7.2
- Sugar: 1.2

76. Cheddar Tarragon Cornbread

Serving: 8 serving(s) | Prep: 10mins | Ready in:

Ingredients

- 1 cup all-purpose flour
- 1 cup yellow cornmeal
- 2 1/2 teaspoons baking powder
- 1/2 teaspoon salt
- 3 tablespoons sugar
- 1/2 cup unsalted butter

- 1 cup buttermilk
- 2 large eggs
- 4 ounces sharp cheddar cheese, grated
- 1 teaspoon chopped fresh tarragon

Direction

- Preheat oven to 425 degrees F. In a medium bowl, combine flour, cornmeal, baking powder, salt, and sugar; set aside.
- Place butter in a 9-inch cast-iron skillet; set in oven until butter melts and begins to brown. In a medium bowl, whisk together buttermilk and eggs. Remove skillet from oven and pour melted butter into buttermilk mixture; whisk to combine and add in Cheddar and tarragon.
- Stir buttermilk mixture into dry ingredients until just combined. Pour into hot skillet and return to oven. Bake until skewer inserted into center tests clean, about 20 minutes.

Nutrition Information

- Calories: 321.2
- Total Carbohydrate: 30.6
- Cholesterol: 99.5
- Sugar: 6.5
- Sodium: 403.8
- Fiber: 1.6
- Protein: 9.1
- Total Fat: 18.4
- Saturated Fat: 10.9

77. Cheese Oatcakes

Serving: 24-48 oatcakes, 8-12 serving(s) | Prep: 10mins | Ready in:

Ingredients

- 4 ounces oatmeal, finely ground
- 4 ounces self-raising flour
- 4 ounces margarine
- 4 ounces cheese, grated
- 1/4 teaspoon salt (optional)

Direction

- Rub margarine or butter into flour and oatmeal.
- Add grated cheese and salt.
- Knead dough well.
- Roll out thinly and cut into rounds, or any shape you choose.
- Bake at 320°F/160°C for 10-15 minutes, or until crisp and golden.

Nutrition Information

- Calories: 253.2
- Total Carbohydrate: 21.5
- Cholesterol: 9.1
- Protein: 6.2
- Total Fat: 15.9
- Sodium: 451.7
- Sugar: 0.2
- Saturated Fat: 4.7
- Fiber: 1.8

78. Cheese Pecan Cocktail Biscuits

Serving: 3 dozen | Prep: 15mins | Ready in:

Ingredients

- 1/2 cup butter
- 1 cup sharp cheddar cheese, grated
- 1 teaspoon salt
- 1/2 teaspoon cayenne pepper
- 1 cup flour
- pecan halves

Direction

- Preheat oven to 350 degrees.
- Cream butter, cheese, salt, and pepper together.
- Beat in flour until smooth.

- Roll into small balls and press a pecan half on each to flatten. Bake 15 minutes at 350 degrees.

Nutrition Information

- Calories: 575.7
- Fiber: 1.2
- Total Carbohydrate: 32.5
- Cholesterol: 120.9
- Total Fat: 43.6
- Saturated Fat: 27.4
- Sodium: 1227.9
- Sugar: 0.4
- Protein: 14

79. Cheesy Biscuits

Serving: 12 biscuits | Prep: 5mins | Ready in:

Ingredients

- 2 1/2 cups Bisquick
- 4 tablespoons butter
- 1 cup of grated cheddar cheese
- 3/4 cup milk
- 1/4 teaspoon garlic powder

Direction

- Mix Bisquick with butter with a fork until small pea-sized chunks form.
- Add heaping cup of cheese with milk and garlic powder.
- Mix by hand until combined, but don't over mix.
- Drop onto ungreased cookie sheet.
- Bake 15 to 17 minutes 400 degrees.

Nutrition Information

- Calories: 188.8
- Total Carbohydrate: 16.7
- Protein: 4.9
- Total Fat: 11.4
- Saturated Fat: 5.8
- Fiber: 0.5
- Sugar: 3
- Sodium: 412.2
- Cholesterol: 22.7

80. Cheesy Treasure Muffins

Serving: 10 muffins, 10 serving(s) | Prep: 10mins | Ready in:

Ingredients

- 1 egg, beaten
- 1 cup milk
- 1/4 cup butter
- 1/4 cup sugar
- 2 cups self rising flour, unsifted
- 1/4 cup green onion, chopped
- 4 slices bacon, cooked, drained and crumbled
- 1/2 cup swiss cheese, shredded
- 1/2 cup sharp cheddar cheese, shredded
- 8 ounces jalapeno jack cheese or 8 ounces colby-monterey jack cheese, cut into 3/4-inch cubes

Direction

- Preheat oven at 400 F.
- In a bowl, mix egg, milk, butter and sugar.
- Slowly stir in flour.
- Fold in the green onions, bacon, Swiss cheese and 1/4 cup cheddar cheese.
- Fill muffin compartments 1/3 full.
- Place one cube of Jalapeno Jack cheese in middle of each muffin compartment on top of batter.
- Continue to fill muffin compartments with batter until 2/3 full.
- Top with remaining cheddar cheese.
- Bake muffins for 15 to 20 minutes or until golden brown.
- Let stand 5 minutes before removing from pan.

- Serve warm.

Nutrition Information

- Calories: 341.7
- Total Fat: 20.6
- Protein: 13.5
- Saturated Fat: 11.5
- Sodium: 612.1
- Fiber: 0.7
- Sugar: 5.4
- Total Carbohydrate: 25.5
- Cholesterol: 74

81. Chef Boy I Be Illinois' Moist And Healthy Cornbread

Serving: 4-6 serving(s) | Prep: 5mins | Ready in:

Ingredients

- 1 cup yellow cornmeal
- 1 cup white flour
- 1/4 cup sugar
- 1/2 teaspoon baking soda
- 1 teaspoon salt
- 1 cup plain nonfat yogurt
- 1/4 cup light sour cream
- 1 egg

Direction

- Preheat oven to 400°F.
- Sift together the corn meal, flour and sugar.
- Mix the baking soda with the yogurt sour cream and egg.
- Combine the yogurt mixture into the corn meal mixture. The batter will be thick, but don't worry.
- Pour mixture into greased (PAM) 8 inch square pan.
- Bake for 20-25 minutes until a toothpick inserted in center comes out clean.

- NOTE: For a more savory corn bread, omit the sugar and try adding any combination of following -- crumbled bacon, shredded cheese, green chilies.

Nutrition Information

- Calories: 344.8
- Saturated Fat: 1.6
- Sugar: 17.6
- Total Carbohydrate: 65.6
- Cholesterol: 59.1
- Sodium: 824.9
- Fiber: 3.1
- Protein: 11.3
- Total Fat: 4.3

82. Chipotle Cheese Mini Muffins

Serving: 36 muffins | Prep: 10mins | Ready in:

Ingredients

- 2 tablespoons sugar
- 1 1/2 cups all-purpose flour
- 1 cup yellow cornmeal
- 1 teaspoon baking soda
- 2 teaspoons baking powder
- 1/2 teaspoon salt
- 1 1/4 cups low-fat buttermilk
- 3 tablespoons canola oil
- 1/2 cup shredded low-fat cheddar cheese
- 3 canned chipotle chiles, rinsed of adobo sauce, chopped fine
- non-stick canola cooking spray

Direction

- Preheat oven to 375 degrees.
- Spray mini-muffin pans with non-stick canola spray.
- Sift together dry ingredients.
- Stir in buttermilk and oil until just blended.
- Do not overstir.

- Fold in cheese and chipotle chilies.
- Fill muffins cups.
- Bake at 375 degrees for 15-20 minutes.
- Best if served warm; can be reheated.

Nutrition Information

- Calories: 51.8
- Cholesterol: 0.7
- Protein: 1.5
- Total Fat: 1.5
- Fiber: 0.5
- Sugar: 1.4
- Total Carbohydrate: 8.1
- Saturated Fat: 0.2
- Sodium: 178.6

83. Choco Low Fat Muffins

Serving: 14 muffins, 14 serving(s) | Prep: 10mins | Ready in:

Ingredients

- 1 1/2 cups flour
- 3/4 cup granulated sugar
- 1/4 cup cocoa
- 2 teaspoons baking powder
- 1 teaspoon baking soda
- 1/2 teaspoon salt
- 2/3 cup low-fat vanilla yogurt
- 2/3 cup nonfat milk
- 1/2 teaspoon vanilla extract
- powdered sugar (optional)

Direction

- Heat oven to 350°F Line muffin cups (2-1/2 inches in diameter) with paper bake cups.
- Stir together flour, granulated sugar, cocoa, baking powder, baking soda and salt in medium bowl; stir in yogurt, milk and vanilla just until combined. Do not beat. Fill muffin cups 2/3 full with batter.
- Bake 15 to 20 minutes or until wooden pick inserted in center comes out clean. Cool slightly in pan on wire rack. Remove from pans. Sprinkle powdered sugar over tops of muffins, if desired. Serve warm.
- Store, covered, at room temperature or freeze in airtight container for longer storage.

Nutrition Information

- Calories: 110.7
- Total Fat: 0.4
- Saturated Fat: 0.1
- Total Carbohydrate: 24.1
- Cholesterol: 0.8
- Protein: 2.6
- Sodium: 238.9
- Fiber: 0.7
- Sugar: 13

84. Chocolate Malted Muffins

Serving: 12 muffins | Prep: 0S | Ready in:

Ingredients

- nonstick cooking spray or paper baking cup
- 1 cup milk (whole, low fat, or non fat)
- 3/4 cup instant malted milk powder
- 2 cups all-purpose flour
- 2 teaspoons baking soda
- 1/2 teaspoon baking powder
- 1/2 teaspoon salt
- 3 ounces unsweetened chocolate, chopped
- 6 tablespoons unsalted butter, room temperature
- 2 large eggs, at room temperature
- 1 cup sugar
- 1 teaspoon vanilla extract

Direction

- Position the rack in the center of the oven and preheat the oven to 400°F

- To prepare the muffin pans, spray the holes and the rims around them with the nonstick spray or line the holes with the paper muffin cups. If using silicone pans, spray as directed, and then set them on a cookie sheet.
- Whisk the milk and malted milk powder in a small bowl until well mixed and the powder has dissolved. Let stand at room temperature for 15 minutes.
- Meanwhile, whisk the flour, baking soda, baking powder and salt in a medium bowl until well mixed. Set aside.
- Place the chocolate and butter in the top of a double boiler set over simmering water. If you don't have a double boiler, place them in a bowl the fits snugly over a small pot of simmering water. Stir constantly until half the butter and chocolate mixture is melted. Remove the top of the double boiler or the bowl from the pot; then continue stirring, away from the heat, until the butter and chocolate are completely smooth. Cool for 5 minutes.
- In a large bowl, whisk the eggs until lightly beaten, then pour in the sugar and continue whisking until the mixture is thick and pale yellow, about 3 minutes. Stir in the vanilla, then the prepared malted milk mixture. Pour in the cooled chocolate mixture in a slow, steady stream, whisking all the while. Finally, using a wooden spoon, stir in the flour mixture, just until moistened.
- Fill the prepared pans three quarters full. Use additional greased pans or small, oven-safe, greased ramekins for any leftover batter. Or save for a second baking. Bake for 20 minutes, or until the muffins have cracked, rounded tops, and a toothpick inserted in the center of a muffin comes out clean.
- Set the pan on a wire rack to cool for 10 minutes. Gently rock each muffin back and forth to release it. Remove them from the pan and let cool on the rack for 5 more minutes. (If storing or freezing, cool completely) Seal in an airtight container or freezer proof bags. Muffins will stay fresh up to 24 hours at room temperature or up to 2 months in the freezer.

Nutrition Information

- Calories: 313.2
- Total Fat: 11.5
- Saturated Fat: 6.7
- Sodium: 387.8
- Fiber: 1.7
- Total Carbohydrate: 49.3
- Sugar: 27.4
- Cholesterol: 53.4
- Protein: 6.3

85. Chocolate Ras Muffin

Serving: 3 muffins | Prep: 5mins | Ready in:

Ingredients

- 2 tablespoons cocoa
- 30 g chocolate protein isolate or 30 g whey protein powder
- 40 g buckwheat groats
- 15 g oatmeal
- 2 (1 g) packets Splenda sugar substitute (optional)
- 1 sliced up banana
- 2 tablespoons plain fat free Greek yogurt or 2 tablespoons vanilla Greek yogurt
- 30 ml unsweetened vanilla almond milk

Direction

- Put everything in a bowl.
- Mix them all up with a spoon until there are no lumps and the content is creamy but not dry (mix for about 3 mins).
- Dump in a muffin tin.
- Bake at 420F for 15-20 minutes.

Nutrition Information

- Calories: 85.2
- Sodium: 8.9

- Sugar: 5.8
- Total Carbohydrate: 17.8
- Cholesterol: 0.2
- Total Fat: 0.9
- Saturated Fat: 0.1
- Fiber: 2.5
- Protein: 2.8

86. Chocolate Soy Low Carb Muffins

Serving: 6 serving(s) | Prep: 5mins | Ready in:

Ingredients

- 3/4 cup soy flour
- 2 eggs
- 1/2 cup cottage cheese
- 1 tablespoon water
- 1 1/2 tablespoons unsweetened cocoa (I prefer Ghirardelli)
- 1 tablespoon vanilla extract
- 1 1/2 tablespoons Splenda sugar substitute

Direction

- Preheat oven to 325.
- Separate egg whites from yolks and beat whites until firm
- In another bowl, mix remaining ingredients Add egg whites and mix.
- Pour mix into 6 greased muffin cups, about 1/2 full.
- Bake at 325 for 20-22 minutes or until knife inserted comes out clean.

Nutrition Information

- Calories: 98.5
- Fiber: 0.5
- Sugar: 0.5
- Sodium: 96
- Saturated Fat: 1.5
- Total Carbohydrate: 4.8

- Cholesterol: 73.1
- Protein: 8.6
- Total Fat: 5

87. Chocolate Wattleseed Biscuits

Serving: 60 biscuits | Prep: 10mins | Ready in:

Ingredients

- 300 g self-raising flour
- 125 g caster sugar
- 25 g cocoa
- 250 g unsalted butter
- 3 teaspoons wattleseed, ground

Direction

- Preheat oven to 170.C.
- Sift flour, cocoa wattleseed.
- Cream butter sugar then work flour into the mix, it will look dry but will eventually bind into a dough.
- Roll into small balls and place well apart on a greased oven tray. Flatten gently with the back of a fork.
- Bake at 170.C for 5 mins then reduce heat to 150.C cook for a further 10 minutes.
- Transfer to a wire rack to cool harden then store in an airtight container.

Nutrition Information

- Calories: 56.6
- Saturated Fat: 2.2
- Fiber: 0.3
- Total Carbohydrate: 6
- Cholesterol: 9
- Total Fat: 3.5
- Sodium: 64
- Sugar: 2.1
- Protein: 0.6

88. Chocolate Zucchini Muffins 1 Point!

Serving: 12 serving(s) | Prep: 5mins | Ready in:

Ingredients

- 3 whole egg whites
- 1/2 cup unsweetened applesauce
- 2/3 cup light brown sugar
- 1 tablespoon vanilla extract
- 1 cup zucchini (shredded)
- 1 1/4 cups whole wheat flour
- 1/4 cup baking cocoa
- 1 teaspoon cinnamon
- 1 teaspoon baking powder

Direction

- Heat oven to 350 degrees and grease 12 muffin cups with non-stick spray.
- Combine all ingredients except zucchini.
- Stir in zucchini.
- Fill the muffin cups and bake for 20 minutes or until muffins test done.

Nutrition Information

- Calories: 107.2
- Sodium: 49.1
- Fiber: 2.3
- Sugar: 13.4
- Saturated Fat: 0.2
- Total Carbohydrate: 24
- Cholesterol: 0
- Protein: 3.1
- Total Fat: 0.6

89. Cilantro Cheddar Drop Biscuits

Serving: 8 serving(s) | Prep: 10mins | Ready in:

Ingredients

- 2 cups flour
- 1 teaspoon salt
- 1/4 teaspoon baking soda
- 3 teaspoons baking powder
- 2 tablespoons shortening
- 1 cup buttermilk (more or less depending on consistency)
- 1 cup cheddar cheese
- 2 green onions, Chopped
- 1 teaspoon granulated garlic
- 2 tablespoons cilantro, Chopped

Direction

- 1. Mix the flour, salt, baking soda, and baking powder together.
- 2. Add the shortening, and cut in until mixture resembles coarse crumbs.
- 3. Stir in the buttermilk.
- 4. Add in remaining ingredients. (Cheese, Onions, Garlic, Cilantro).
- 5. Preheat oven to 425°, drop by heaping tablespoonfuls onto greased baking sheet.
- 6. Bake for 10-12 minutes, or until a toothpick inserted comes out clean.

Nutrition Information

- Calories: 214.5
- Total Fat: 8.5
- Cholesterol: 16.1
- Sodium: 587.5
- Fiber: 1
- Sugar: 1.8
- Total Carbohydrate: 26.4
- Protein: 7.9
- Saturated Fat: 4

90. Cinnamon Cornbread

Serving: 9-12 pieces of cornbread, 5-6 serving(s) | Prep: 20mins | Ready in:

Ingredients

- 1/4 cup canola oil
- 1 1/4 cups stone-ground cornmeal
- 3/4 cup unbleached all-purpose flour
- 1 teaspoon baking soda
- 1 1/2 teaspoons baking powder
- 1/4 teaspoon sea salt
- 3 -4 tablespoons sugar
- 2 eggs, beaten
- 1 cup 2% low-fat milk
- 1 teaspoon cinnamon
- 1/2 teaspoon allspice
- 1/8 teaspoon ground cloves
- 1/4 teaspoon vanilla (optional)
- rose water, to taste (optional)
- rosemary, to taste (optional)
- peppermint oil, to taste (optional)

Direction

- Preheat oven to 400°F.
- Oil a 9x9 inch baking pan. Other sizes could probably work too, just watch your baking time so it doesn't burn.
- Stir all dry ingredients together in a large bowl.
- Stir all wet ingredients together in a medium bowl.
- Stir the wet and dry ingredients together. Keep the batter a bit lumpy.
- Pour batter into pan and sprinkle some extra cinnamon on top, swirling it into the batter slightly.
- Bake for 20-26 minutes until done. The center should spring back when touched. Let it sit 5-10 minutes before cutting, if you can resist!

Nutrition Information

- Calories: 360.7
- Saturated Fat: 2.2
- Sodium: 536.4
- Protein: 8.6
- Total Fat: 15.2
- Fiber: 3
- Sugar: 10.4
- Total Carbohydrate: 48.6
- Cholesterol: 88.5

91. Cinnamon Raisin Muffins

Serving: 24 mini muffins, 24 serving(s) | Prep: 15mins | Ready in:

Ingredients

- 2 cups all-purpose flour
- 3 teaspoons baking powder
- 1/2 teaspoon salt
- 3/4 cup white sugar
- 1 egg
- 1 cup milk
- 1/4 cup vegetable oil
- 1/2 teaspoon cinnamon
- 65 g raisins

Direction

- 1. Preheat oven to 400 degrees F (200 degrees C).
- 2. Stir together the flour, baking powder, salt, cinnamon and sugar and raisins in a large bowl. Make a well in the center. In a small bowl or 2 cup measuring cup, beat egg with a fork. Stir in milk and oil. Pour all at once into the well in the flour mixture. Mix quickly and lightly with a fork until moistened, but do not beat. The batter will be lumpy. Pour the batter into paper lined muffin pan cups.
- 3. If you're making mini muffins, bake it for at least 12 minutes. If making large muffins, bake it for at least 20-25 minutes.

Nutrition Information

- Calories: 105.5
- Cholesterol: 10.2
- Protein: 1.8
- Total Fat: 3

- Saturated Fat: 0.6
- Sodium: 102.4
- Fiber: 0.5
- Sugar: 8.9
- Total Carbohydrate: 18.4

92. Cinnamon Raisin Scones

Serving: 8 scones, 8 serving(s) | Prep: 15mins | Ready in:

Ingredients

- 1 3/4 cups whole wheat flour
- 3 tablespoons sugar (I use splenda granular)
- 1 tablespoon baking powder
- 1 teaspoon ground cinnamon
- 1/2 teaspoon salt
- 2 tablespoons butter
- 2 tablespoons applesauce
- 1/2 cup 1% low-fat milk (I use fat free milk)
- 1 egg (I use liquid egg whites)
- 1/3 cup raisins (or dried cranberries)
- 3 tablespoons whole wheat flour

Direction

- Preheat oven to 425 degrees.
- In a medium-sized mixing bowl, measure 1 3/4 cups flour, 3 tablespoons sugar, baking powder, cinnamon and salt. Mix together with a large spoon.
- Melt butter and place in a medium bowl with the applesauce. Add milk, egg and raisins. Stir until ingredients are blended.
- Add wet ingredients to flour mixture. Stir until dough forms into a ball.
- Sprinkle the 3 tablespoons flour on a flat surface. Flour your hands well and move dough from bowl to surface. Knead the dough by using the heel of your hand to push the dough away from you. Then with your hands, pull the dough back toward you, folding over as you pull it. Repeat this for about 1 minute.
- Place the kneaded dough on an ungreased cookie sheet or pizza pan. Pat the dough into an 8" circle. With a knife or pizza cutter, cut the dough into 8 wedges.
- Bake for 15-20 minutes or until golden brown.

Nutrition Information

- Calories: 180.4
- Total Fat: 4.2
- Sodium: 320.7
- Total Carbohydrate: 32.8
- Saturated Fat: 2.2
- Fiber: 4
- Sugar: 9.3
- Cholesterol: 34.8
- Protein: 5.5

93. Cinnamon Scones

Serving: 12 serving(s) | Prep: 15mins | Ready in:

Ingredients

- 1 cup sour cream
- 1 teaspoon baking soda
- 4 cups all-purpose flour
- 1 cup white sugar
- 2 teaspoons baking powder
- 1/4 teaspoon cream of tartar
- 1 teaspoon salt
- 1 cup butter
- 1 egg
- 4 teaspoons cinnamon
- For dusting
- sugar
- cinnamon

Direction

- Preheat oven to 350 F degrees.
- Spray two baking sheets with non-stick cooking spray.
- Combine sour cream and baking soda in a small bowl.

- Combine flour, sugar, baking powder, cream of tartar and salt in another bowl.
- Cut in butter until mixture resembles fine breadcrumbs.
- Combine egg with sour cream mixture, add cinnamon.
- Gently stir into flour mixture until moistened.
- IMPORTANT: knead dough briefly, no more than 10 times.
- Divide dough into two, place on baking sheet and pat into 3/4 inch thickness.
- Cut each round into 6 wedge-shaped pieces.
- Move scones so they are not touching (at least 3 inches), dust with sugar and cinnamon.
- Bake 15-20 minutes or until golden brown.

Nutrition Information

- Calories: 397.4
- Fiber: 1.6
- Sugar: 17.5
- Total Carbohydrate: 50
- Cholesterol: 66.1
- Total Fat: 19.9
- Saturated Fat: 12.1
- Sodium: 516.6
- Protein: 5.4

94. Cleaned Up Scottish Oatcakes

Serving: 18 Oatcakes, 9 serving(s) | Prep: 15mins | Ready in:

Ingredients

- 1 cup slow cook oats
- 1 cup whole wheat flour
- 1/2 teaspoon baking soda
- 1/4 teaspoon salt
- 1/2 cup coconut oil
- 2-3 tablespoons water, ice cold

Direction

- Heat oven to 375.
- Mix the dry ingredients, then cut the shortening in until it resembles fine crumbs. (I gave up on this and just smooshed it with my hands.) Add water, 1 tablespoon at a time, until mixture forms a stiff dough when you press it together. (Alternatively, you can mix this in your food processor).
- On lightly wheat-floured surface, roll the dough out to about 1/8-inch thick. If needed, use ice water as "glue" to patch it together- It might fall apart a little. Cut into rounds with a large cookie cutter or the top of a glass about 2 1/2" in diameter. Or you can cut it into squares with a knife. Place on an ungreased baking sheet.
- Bake until the oatcakes start to brown, about 12-15 minutes. Cool a bit on a wire rack, if your gang will wait that long.
- To serve, top with whatever you find in your kitchen. These are not sweet, so they make a great base for sweeter toppings like jelly and honey. Other toppings we've use are peanut butter, butter, sliced fruit, cream cheese and coconut. I think we even used chocolate chips a time or two. Use your imagination!
- Per serving (2 oatcakes): 183 calories, 3g protein, 16g carbohydrate, 12g healthy fats, 2.5g fiber, 135mg sodium.

Nutrition Information

- Calories: 217.2
- Sugar: 0.1
- Total Carbohydrate: 21.1
- Cholesterol: 0
- Protein: 4.7
- Total Fat: 13.6
- Saturated Fat: 10.7
- Sodium: 135.2
- Fiber: 3.3

95. Coconut Flour Agave Nectar Muffins

Serving: 6 muffins, 6 serving(s) | Prep: 10mins | Ready in:

Ingredients

- 1/4 cup coconut flour
- 3 eggs
- 1/4 teaspoon vanilla
- 1/4 teaspoon salt
- 2 tablespoons coconut oil
- 2 tablespoons coconut milk
- 2 tablespoons agave nectar
- 1/4 teaspoon baking powder
- 1 pinch stevia

Direction

- Mix wet ingredients, then add dry sifted ingredients until smooth. Bake at 400 degrees for 15 minute.

Nutrition Information

- Calories: 85.3
- Cholesterol: 93
- Fiber: 0
- Total Carbohydrate: 0.4
- Sugar: 0.1
- Protein: 3.2
- Total Fat: 8
- Saturated Fat: 5.7
- Sodium: 148.2

96. Coconut And Raspberry Muffins

Serving: 12 muffins | Prep: 10mins | Ready in:

Ingredients

- 2 cups flour
- 4 teaspoons baking powder
- 3/4 cup desiccated coconut
- 1/4 cup soft brown sugar
- 250 g frozen raspberries, slightly thawed (reserve 12 for topping)
- 1/4 cup white sugar
- 1 teaspoon vanilla essence (vanilla extract)
- 60 g butter, melted
- 2 eggs
- 1 cup milk
- 4 tablespoons shredded coconut, for topping

Direction

- Preheat oven to 200°C. Lightly grease 12 muffin tins.
- Sift together flour and baking powder into a bowl. Stir in coconut and soft brown sugar.
- Place raspberries in a bowl and cover with white sugar.
- In another bowl lightly whisk together the vanilla, melted butter, eggs and milk. Pour over raspberries.
- Fold egg mixture into dry ingredients and stir quickly to combine.
- Spoon mixture into prepared muffin tins, sprinkle with coconut shreds and press one raspberry into the center of each muffin.
- Bake for 12 - 15 minutes or until muffins spring back when lightly pressed.

Nutrition Information

- Calories: 224.8
- Sodium: 190.5
- Saturated Fat: 5.2
- Fiber: 1.8
- Sugar: 16.1
- Total Carbohydrate: 34.5
- Cholesterol: 48.8
- Protein: 4.3
- Total Fat: 8

97. Coffee Muffins

Serving: 16 large | Prep: 10mins | Ready in:

Ingredients

- 3 cups sifted cake flour
- 4 teaspoons baking powder
- 3/4 cup brown sugar
- 1/2 teaspoon salt
- 1 cup pecans, broken
- 1 egg
- 1 1/4 cups strong cold coffee
- 2 tablespoons shortening, melted

Direction

- Sift dry ingredients together and add nuts.
- Beat egg.
- Add coffee and shortening and add to dry ingredients.
- Mix only enough to dampen all the flour.
- Bake in greased muffin pans at 400 for 20-25 minutes.

Nutrition Information

- Calories: 198.6
- Protein: 3.1
- Saturated Fat: 0.9
- Fiber: 1.1
- Total Carbohydrate: 31.4
- Cholesterol: 13.2
- Total Fat: 7
- Sodium: 172.5
- Sugar: 10.3

98. Coffee Shop Cornbread Muffins

Serving: 10-12 Muffins | Prep: 10mins | Ready in:

Ingredients

- 1 1/4 cups yellow cornmeal
- 1 cup unsifted flour
- 1/3 cup sugar
- 1 teaspoon baking soda
- 1/2 teaspoon salt
- 1/3 cup packed brown sugar
- 1 egg
- 1 cup buttermilk
- 3/4 cup oil

Direction

- In a bowl, stir together corn meal, flour, sugar, baking soda, salt and brown sugar.
- In a second bowl, whisk egg with buttermilk (or sour milk) and oil.
- Add liquid ingredients to dry ingredients all at once, stirring just until blended.
- Spoon into well-greased muffin pans, filling about ¾ full.
- Bake in a preheated 425°F oven for 20 minutes or until a golden brown.
- Enjoy warm, cooled to room temperature or split and toasted.

Nutrition Information

- Calories: 315.8
- Saturated Fat: 2.5
- Sugar: 15.1
- Total Carbohydrate: 36.3
- Protein: 4
- Total Fat: 17.7
- Sodium: 282.7
- Fiber: 1.4
- Cholesterol: 19.6

99. Corey's Biscuits

Serving: 8 serving(s) | Prep: 10mins | Ready in:

Ingredients

- 2 cups flour
- 2 teaspoons baking powder
- 1/2 teaspoon baking soda
- 2 tablespoons sugar
- 1/4 cup butter

- 1 cup milk or 1 cup half-and-half (or half cup of each)

Direction

- Mix flour, baking powder, baking soda and sugar.
- Cut in butter.
- Add milk.
- Do not overmix and pat into biscuit shapes.
- Bake at 375 for 20 minutes.

Nutrition Information

- Calories: 196.9
- Total Carbohydrate: 28.7
- Protein: 4.3
- Total Fat: 7.2
- Sodium: 225.9
- Fiber: 0.8
- Sugar: 3.2
- Cholesterol: 19.5
- Saturated Fat: 4.4

100. Corn 'n Blueberry Muffins

Serving: 5-6 Muffins, 6 serving(s) | Prep: 15mins | Ready in:

Ingredients

- 1/2 cup all-purpose flour
- 1/2 cup cornmeal
- 1/2 teaspoon baking soda
- 1/2 teaspoon sea salt
- 1 extra large egg
- 5 tablespoons agave syrup
- 1/2 cup yogurt
- 1/2 cup mayonnaise
- 3/4 cup fresh blueberries

Direction

- In a small bowl, combine the flour, cornmeal, baking soda and salt.
- In another bowl, beat egg with agave syrup, yogurt and mayonnaise.
- Sift dry ingredients into the egg mixture and stir just until moistened.
- Spray a large 6-cup muffin tin with butter spray and fill 2/3 full.
- Press fresh blueberries into each cup and stir lightly to blend.
- Bake at 400F for 15 minutes or until a toothpick comes out clean.
- Cool for 5 minutes before removing from pan.
- Serve with softened butter.

Nutrition Information

- Calories: 186
- Total Carbohydrate: 24.1
- Cholesterol: 38.8
- Protein: 4
- Fiber: 1.5
- Sugar: 4.2
- Total Fat: 8.5
- Saturated Fat: 1.7
- Sodium: 463.1

101. Corn Grits Cornbread

Serving: 9 serving(s) | Prep: 5mins | Ready in:

Ingredients

- 1/2 cup cornmeal (regular)
- 1/2 cup cornmeal, coarsely ground (corn grits or polenta)
- 1 cup flour
- 2 teaspoons baking powder
- 1 tablespoon sugar
- 1 teaspoon salt
- 1 cup buttermilk (or put 1 Tablespoon vinegar in your measuring cup and fill to 1 cup with milk)
- 1/2 teaspoon baking soda

- 2 eggs
- 1/2 cup butter, melted

Direction

- (Make "buttermilk" if you're going to do that, so it can sit a bit and do whatever it does that makes it buttermilky.).
- Preheat oven to 425°F.
- Combine the dry ingredients (except the soda).
- Stir the baking soda into the buttermilk and add that to the dry ingredients.
- Add eggs and melted butter. Stir together and pour into a 9x9 pan.
- Bake for 20 minutes.

Nutrition Information

- Calories: 223.2
- Saturated Fat: 7.1
- Sodium: 530.8
- Sugar: 2.9
- Total Carbohydrate: 24.1
- Protein: 4.9
- Total Fat: 12.2
- Fiber: 1.4
- Cholesterol: 75.2

102. Cornbread Muffins

Serving: 12 serving(s) | Prep: 10mins | Ready in:

Ingredients

- 3/4 cup cornmeal
- 1 cup all-purpose flour
- 1/4 cup white sugar
- 1 tablespoon baking powder
- 1/4 teaspoon salt
- 1 egg, lightly beaten
- 1 cup 1% low-fat milk
- 1/4 cup unsalted butter, melted

Direction

- Preheat oven to 425 degrees.
- Spray muffin tin with non-stick spray or line with paper muffin cups.
- Combine cornmeal, flour, sugar, baking powder and salt.
- Stir well.
- Combine beaten egg, milk and melted butter (if using normal butter add less salt).
- Stir into the dry mixture and combine just until blended.
- Chopped jalapenos (from a tin) can also be added, as can chopped red pepper and/or tinned corn kernels.
- Scoop batter into prepared muffin pans.
- Sprinkle cheddar cheese on top of muffins before baking if desired.
- Bake for 20-25 minutes.

Nutrition Information

- Calories: 130.6
- Sugar: 5.3
- Protein: 3
- Total Fat: 4.8
- Saturated Fat: 2.7
- Sodium: 157.5
- Fiber: 0.8
- Total Carbohydrate: 19.3
- Cholesterol: 26.7

103. Cornbread And Basil Muffins With Fresh Corn

Serving: 24 muffins | Prep: 10mins | Ready in:

Ingredients

- 1 1/2 cups low-fat buttermilk
- 3 large eggs
- 1/3 cup fresh basil
- 2 cups yellow cornmeal
- 1 cup all-purpose flour
- 1/2 cup sugar

- 4 teaspoons baking powder
- 1 teaspoon salt
- 1/2 cup light butter, diced
- 1 1/2 cups corn

Direction

- Preheat oven to 400°F Brush muffin pans with butter.
- Chop basil as finely as possible. Whisk buttermilk, eggs, and basil in large bowl.
- Blend cornmeal, flour, sugar, and baking powder in food processor for 10 seconds.
- Dice 1 stick of butter (i.e., 1/2 cup) and blend with dry ingredients until coarse meal forms.
- Stir ingredients from food processor into buttermilk mixture, mixing in a little bit at a time. Make sure clumps of butter have been dissolved. Add corn kernels and stir thoroughly.
- Transfer mixture to muffin pans.
- Bake cornbread until golden on top and toothpick inserted into center comes out clean (about 15 minutes). Cool 20 minutes. Serve warm or at room temperature.

Nutrition Information

- Calories: 121
- Protein: 3.1
- Total Fat: 4
- Saturated Fat: 2
- Fiber: 1.1
- Sugar: 5.4
- Sodium: 207.9
- Total Carbohydrate: 18.9
- Cholesterol: 29

104. Cornmeal (Cornbread) Mix

Serving: 40 muffins, 40 serving(s) | Prep: 10mins | Ready in:

Ingredients

- 4 cups flour
- 4 cups cornmeal
- 1 1/2 cups nonfat dry milk powder
- 2/3 cup granulated sugar (optional)
- 1/4 cup baking powder
- 2 teaspoons salt
- 1 1/2 cups shortening

Direction

- Sift dry ingredients together until well mixed. Cut in fat until well blended. Place in a glass jar. Keep tightly closed in a cool place. Mixture will keep for 1 to 6 months on the shelf in dry weather. In hot and humid weather, store in the refrigerator.
- Cornmeal Muffins-Grease 8 medium-size muffin cups. Combine 2-1/4 cups Cornmeal Mix, 2/3 cup water and 1 beaten egg. Stir just enough to moisten dry ingredients. Fill muffin cups 2/3 full. Bake at 425 degrees F for about 20 minutes. Makes 8.
- Cornmeal Biscuits-Add about 1/2 cup water to 2 cups Cornmeal Mix to make a soft dough. Drop by tablespoonfuls onto a greased baking sheet. Bake at 425 degrees F for 12 minutes. Makes 12 biscuits.
- Cornbread-Combine 4 1/2 cups Cornmeal Mix, 2 beaten eggs and 1 1/3 cups water. Stir just enough to moisten dry ingredients. Pour into a greased pan, about 8 inches square. Bake at 425 degrees F for about 25 minutes. Serves 12.
- Blueberry Cornbread: Add 1 cup fresh or partially-thawed frozen blueberries to Cornbread batter and mix gently. Bake as directed.
- Cheese Cornbread: After turning Cornbread batter into pan, sprinkle with shredded Cheddar cheese and sesame seed. Bake as directed.

Nutrition Information

- Calories: 174.5

- Sugar: 2.5
- Cholesterol: 0.9
- Total Fat: 8.3
- Sodium: 253.8
- Fiber: 1.2
- Saturated Fat: 2
- Total Carbohydrate: 21.6
- Protein: 3.9

105. Cracker Barrel Old Country Store Biscuits

Serving: 10 biscuits | Prep: 15mins | Ready in:

Ingredients

- 2 1/4 cups Bisquick
- 2/3 cup buttermilk
- 1 teaspoon sugar
- 1 tablespoon butter, melted
- melted butter, for brushing

Direction

- Preheat oven to 450°F.
- Mix the Bisquick, buttermilk and sugar together in a bowl.
- Add the melted butter into the batter.
- Stir until a soft dough forms.
- Turn out onto a well-floured work surface.
- Knead 20 times (this is a very forgiving dough), and don't be afraid to get additional flour into the dough.
- Roll 1/2 thick, or thicker if you prefer towering biscuits.
- Cut out into 2" rounds (or your preferred size).
- Place close together on an ungreased baking sheet.
- Brush tops with melted butter.
- Bake for 8 to 10 minutes; I usually find 8 minutes is enough.
- When you remove the biscuits from the oven, brush the tops with melted butter again.

Nutrition Information

- Calories: 141.6
- Saturated Fat: 2
- Total Carbohydrate: 19.4
- Cholesterol: 4.3
- Protein: 2.9
- Total Fat: 5.7
- Sugar: 4.6
- Sodium: 318.8
- Fiber: 0.6

106. Cran Bran Muffins

Serving: 12 muffins | Prep: 15mins | Ready in:

Ingredients

- 1 1/2 cups natural bran, 100% natural (not All-Bran)
- 1 cup low-fat buttermilk (or 1 cup fat-free milk mixed with 1 TBS of lemon juice)
- 1 cup all-purpose flour
- 1 teaspoon baking powder
- 1 teaspoon baking soda
- 1/2 teaspoon salt
- 1/2 teaspoon vanilla
- 1/2 cup dried cranberries
- 1 large egg
- 2/3 cup brown sugar, lightly packed
- 1/3 cup unsweetened apple butter

Direction

- Preheat oven to 375 and grease 12-cup muffin pan (or use paper liners).
- Mix buttermilk with bran and set aside.
- Mix together apple butter, brown sugar, vanilla and egg.
- Add to bran mixture.
- Sift together flour, baking soda, baking powder and salt.
- Add to wet ingredients.
- Stir just until combined.
- Fold in dried cranberries.

- Divide batter into 12 muffin cups and bake for 12-15 minutes, or until they test clean.
- Cool for 5 minutes in pan, then completely cool upside down on wire rack. (This prevents soggy bottoms!).

Nutrition Information

- Calories: 133.9
- Total Fat: 1.1
- Sodium: 283.7
- Cholesterol: 18.4
- Saturated Fat: 0.3
- Fiber: 2.8
- Sugar: 16.9
- Total Carbohydrate: 30.4
- Protein: 3.3

107. Cranberry Walnut Scones

Serving: 12 Scones, 12 serving(s) | Prep: 15mins | Ready in:

Ingredients

- 2 cups all-purpose flour
- 1/4 teaspoon baking soda
- 1 tablespoon baking powder
- 1/3 cup sugar
- 2 tablespoons margarine
- 1/3 cup dried cranberries
- 1 tablespoon vanilla extract
- 1 cup buttermilk, nonfat
- cooking spray
- 3 tablespoons walnuts, chopped
- 1 1/2 teaspoons sugar

Direction

- Pre-heat oven to 400°F. Coat baking sheets with cooking spray.
- Combine flour, baking powder, baking soda, and sugar in a medium bowl; cut in margarine with a pastry blender until mixture resembles coarse meal. Stir in cranberries.
- Add buttermilk and vanilla, stirring with a fork until dry ingredients are moistened.
- Spoon 2 heaping tablespoonfuls of dough, 2 inches apart, onto baking sheets coated with cooking spray. Sprinkle evenly with walnuts and 1 ½ teaspoons sugar.
- Bake at 400F for 15 to 17 minutes or until golden. Makes 12 scones.

Nutrition Information

- Calories: 141.1
- Total Carbohydrate: 23.9
- Total Fat: 3.5
- Saturated Fat: 0.6
- Sodium: 161.2
- Fiber: 0.8
- Sugar: 7.4
- Cholesterol: 0.8
- Protein: 3.1

108. Cranberry Zucchini Muffins

Serving: 12 muffins, 12 serving(s) | Prep: 0S | Ready in:

Ingredients

- 1 3/4 cups all-purpose flour
- 1/2 teaspoon baking powder
- 1/2 teaspoon baking soda
- 1 teaspoon ground cinnamon
- 1/4 teaspoon salt
- 2 large eggs
- 1/2 cup sugar
- 1/2 cup brown sugar
- 1/2 cup applesauce
- 1 teaspoon vanilla extract
- 1 cup grated zucchini
- 1/2 cup cranberries, chopped

Direction

- Preheat oven to 375°F. Grease muffin tin; set aside.
- In a medium bowl, whisk together the flour, baking soda, baking powder, baking soda, cinnamon and salt; set aside.
- In a large bowl, whisk together the eggs, sugars, applesauce and vanilla. Stir in the zucchini.
- Add the flour mixture to the wet ingredients, and stir to combine; do not overmix. Using a rubber spatula fold in the cranberries. Divide the batter evenly among the 12 cups.
- Bake, rotating the pan halfway through, until the muffins are golden, 25 to 30 minutes. Transfer the pan to a wire rack to cool for 10 minutes. Turn the muffins on their sides in their cups, and cool.
- Bread Variation: Follow instructions for muffins, transferring batter to a 9x5 loaf pan, buttered or sprayed with non-stick spray. Bake at 375 F, rotating the pan halfway through, 45-50 minutes. Transfer to wire rack to cool before serving.

Nutrition Information

- Calories: 158.6
- Total Carbohydrate: 34.4
- Total Fat: 1.1
- Saturated Fat: 0.3
- Sodium: 135.8
- Fiber: 1
- Sugar: 17.6
- Cholesterol: 35.2
- Protein: 3.1

109. Cranberry Orange Muffins (Diabetic Friendly)

Serving: 12 muffins, 12 serving(s) | Prep: 5mins | Ready in:

Ingredients

- 3/4 cup Splenda granular
- 1 cup coarsley cut cranberries
- 1 cup white flour
- 1 cup whole wheat flour
- 1 1/2 teaspoons baking powder
- 1/2 teaspoon salt
- 1/2 teaspoon baking soda
- 1/2 cup chopped walnuts (optional)
- 1 beaten egg
- 3/4 cup orange juice
- 3 tablespoons oil
- 1 teaspoon grated orange peel

Direction

- Combine cranberries and sugar while sifting dry ingredients together -- then add and stir into dry ingredients.
- Combine egg, juice and oil and grated peel and add to dry ingredients until just moistened.
- Pour batter into 12 muffin cups, lightly sprayed or into paper muffin liners (or a loaf pan).
- Bake muffins at 375 degrees for 25".
- Bake loaf at 350 degrees for 50".

Nutrition Information

- Calories: 119.2
- Total Carbohydrate: 18
- Cholesterol: 15.5
- Protein: 3.1
- Total Fat: 4.2
- Saturated Fat: 0.6
- Sodium: 201.4
- Fiber: 1.8
- Sugar: 1.7

110. Crazy Biscuits

Serving: 20 serving(s) | Prep: 10mins | Ready in:

Ingredients

- 2 cups flour
- 1/2 teaspoon salt
- 1/2 teaspoon cream of tartar
- 4 teaspoons baking powder
- 2 teaspoons sugar
- 1/2 cup shortening
- 2/3 cup milk

Direction

- Sift dry ingredients into a bowl.
- Cut in shortening until mixture resembles coarse crumbs.
- Add milk and stir until dough follows fork around bowl.
- Knead slightly.
- Pat out on lightly floured board and cut.
- Bake on an ungreased cookie sheet at 450°F for 10 to 20 minutes, or until brown.
- TO REHEAT leftover biscuits, wrap in foil and heat in a 300°F oven for 10 minutes.
- Open foil half through heating if you want them crisp.

Nutrition Information

- Calories: 98.2
- Sugar: 0.5
- Total Carbohydrate: 10.6
- Saturated Fat: 1.5
- Sodium: 135
- Fiber: 0.3
- Cholesterol: 1.1
- Protein: 1.6
- Total Fat: 5.5

111. Crustless Breakfast Quiche Muffins

Serving: 12 serving(s) | Prep: 15mins | Ready in:

Ingredients

- 3 eggs
- 1 1/2 cups milk
- 1/2 cup baking mix
- 12 ounces sausage
- 1/2 cup cheddar cheese, shredded

Direction

- Preheat oven to 350.
- Brown sausage, breaking with a spoon. Drain well.
- Mix egg, milk and baking mix. Season with salt and pepper.
- Divide egg mixture between 12 greased muffin tins.
- Divide sausage between muffin tins and cover with cheese.
- Bake 15-20 minutes or until tooth pick inserted comes out clean.
- Freeze left over muffins in single serving zip top bags. To reheat, place frozen muffins in microwave for approximately 60 seconds.

Nutrition Information

- Calories: 169.9
- Fiber: 0.1
- Total Carbohydrate: 5.6
- Cholesterol: 72.3
- Total Fat: 12.8
- Sodium: 374.2
- Sugar: 0.7
- Protein: 7.6
- Saturated Fat: 5.1

112. Custard Powder Biscuits (Cookies)

Serving: 36 cookies | Prep: 10mins | Ready in:

Ingredients

- 125 g butter, softened
- 1 cup caster sugar
- 1 egg, at room temperature

- 1/2 teaspoon vanilla essence
- 1 1/2 cups self-raising flour
- 1/2 cup custard powder
- 80 g white chocolate, roughly chopped

Direction

- Preheat oven to 180C and line 2 baking trays with baking paper.
- Using an electric mixer, cream butter and sugar until light and fluffy. Add egg and vanilla and beat until well combined.
- Sift flour and custard powder together over butter mixture. Add white chocolate and stir until mixture forms a soft dough.
- Roll tablespoonfuls of mixture into balls and place on prepared trays, allowing room for spreading. Using a fork, press dough to flatten slightly.
- Bake for 10 to 12 minutes or until golden. Stand on trays for 5 minutes then transfer to a wire rack to cool.

Nutrition Information

- Calories: 78.8
- Total Fat: 3.7
- Fiber: 0.1
- Total Carbohydrate: 10.8
- Protein: 0.8
- Saturated Fat: 2.3
- Sodium: 94.8
- Sugar: 6.9
- Cholesterol: 13.1

113. Dad's Breakfast Egg Muffins

Serving: 12 Muffins, 12 serving(s) | Prep: 10mins | Ready in:

Ingredients

- 7 large eggs
- 3 sausage patties (chopped) or 6 slices bacon (chopped)
- 1/2 cup cheddar cheese (shredded)
- 1 small onion (chopped)
- 1/4 cup bell pepper (chopped)
- 1/4 cup tomatoes (chopped)
- 1/8 cup mushroom (chopped)
- 2 slices bread (1/4-inch cubed)
- 1/2 teaspoon salt
- 1/4 teaspoon pepper
- 1/4 teaspoon onion powder
- 1/4 teaspoon garlic powder

Direction

- Pre heat oven to 400 degrees.
- In a large bowl mix cheese, veggies, eggs and meat. Mix with a hand mixer until frothy.
- Add Spices, continue to mix.
- Fold in bread.
- Spoon mixture into greased muffin pan.
- Cook for 20 min and enjoy.

Nutrition Information

- Calories: 76.1
- Total Fat: 4.5
- Sodium: 189.5
- Sugar: 0.8
- Cholesterol: 113.4
- Saturated Fat: 1.9
- Fiber: 0.3
- Total Carbohydrate: 3.4
- Protein: 5.3

114. Dainty Crusty Biscuits

Serving: 18 bisquits, 18 serving(s) | Prep: 15mins | Ready in:

Ingredients

- 2 cups all-purpose flour
- 2 1/2 teaspoons baking powder

- 1/2 teaspoon salt
- 3/4 cup skim milk
- 1/3 cup vegetable oil

Direction

- Combine flour, baking powder and salt in a medium mixing bowl, gradually add milk and oil, stirring until just moistened.
- Turn dough out onto a lightly floured surface, and knead lightly 2 or 3 times.
- Pat dough to a 1/2-inch thickness, and cut with a floured 1 3/4-inch bisquit cutter.
- Arrange bisquits with sides lightly touching on an ungreased baking sheet.
- Bake at 450 degrees for 12 to 15 minutes.

Nutrition Information

- Calories: 90.7
- Total Fat: 4.2
- Saturated Fat: 0.6
- Sugar: 0
- Cholesterol: 0.2
- Sodium: 121.3
- Fiber: 0.4
- Total Carbohydrate: 11.3
- Protein: 1.8

115. Date Pineapple Breakfast Muffins

Serving: 24 32, 24 serving(s) | Prep: 10mins | Ready in:

Ingredients

- 2 eggs
- 1 egg white
- 1 (20 ounce) can crushed pineapple
- 1/2 cup apple butter
- 1/2 cup canola oil
- 2/3 cup dried dates
- 1/3 cup raisins
- 2 teaspoons vanilla extract
- 1 cup white sugar
- 2 teaspoons cinnamon
- 1 teaspoon salt
- 3 cups white flour
- 1 cup oats
- 2 teaspoons baking soda
- 1 1/4 teaspoons baking powder
- 1/2 cup pecans (optional)

Direction

- In a large mixing bowl, mix eggs, pineapple with undrained juice, apple, butter, oil, sugar, vanilla, dates, raisins, oatmeals, cinnamon, and salt.
- Then fold in flour, baking powder, baking soda and nuts if you used them.
- Mix with wooden spoon until combined well.
- Grease muffin pans with nonstick spray.
- Scoop out 1/3 cup of batter into standard muffin pans. Bake in 350 degree oven for about 20 minutes.
- Depending on your batter scoops you should get about 24-32 muffins.

Nutrition Information

- Calories: 204.8
- Total Fat: 5.6
- Sugar: 17.7
- Total Carbohydrate: 35.7
- Protein: 3.7
- Saturated Fat: 0.6
- Sodium: 230.9
- Fiber: 1.9
- Cholesterol: 15.5

116. Deception Muffins

Serving: 12 serving(s) | Prep: 5mins | Ready in:

Ingredients

- 2 cups flour

- 2 teaspoons baking powder
- 1/2 teaspoon salt
- 2 eggs
- 1 teaspoon vegetable oil
- 1/4 cup honey
- 1 1/2 cups milk or 1 1/2 cups water
- 2 cups shredded cooked leftover vegetables

Direction

- Preheat the oven to 400 degrees and line muffin tins with cupcake liners.
- Combine the dry ingredients.
- Mix the wet ingredients.
- Combine wet and dry ingredients; stir veggies into mix.
- Put into 12 muffin cups.
- Bake 20-22 minutes.

Nutrition Information

- Calories: 132.8
- Saturated Fat: 1
- Protein: 4.2
- Sodium: 184.7
- Fiber: 0.6
- Sugar: 5.9
- Total Carbohydrate: 23.4
- Cholesterol: 39.5
- Total Fat: 2.5

117. Delicious Low Fat/Low Cal Cornbread

Serving: 10 serving(s) | Prep: 5mins | Ready in:

Ingredients

- 1/4 cup whole wheat flour
- 1/4 cup white flour
- 3 tablespoons sugar
- 1/2 teaspoon salt (or less)
- 1 cup yellow cornmeal
- 2 egg whites
- 3/4 cup skim milk
- 1/3 cup unsweetened applesauce

Direction

- Preheat oven to 425°; grease pan and set in oven to preheat.
- Mix together dry ingredients. Beat together egg, milk, applesauce, and add to dry ingredients.
- Pour into hot pan and bake for 20 minutes.
- My dad likes it with butter, right out of the oven or later when it's cool, and I like it with homemade strawberry jelly. Enjoy!

Nutrition Information

- Calories: 94.8
- Saturated Fat: 0.1
- Cholesterol: 0.4
- Protein: 3.2
- Sugar: 4.7
- Total Carbohydrate: 19.7
- Total Fat: 0.6
- Sodium: 142.7
- Fiber: 1.4

118. Delicious Low Cal Banana Muffins :)

Serving: 10-12 serving(s) | Prep: 10mins | Ready in:

Ingredients

- 2 cups all-purpose flour
- 2 tablespoons baking powder
- 1 teaspoon baking soda
- 1/4 teaspoon kosher salt
- 2 cups bananas, mashed
- 2 eggs
- 1 teaspoon vanilla extract
- 1/2 cup sugar
- 1/2 cup applesauce

- 1 cup chocolate chips (Optional, but Recommended)

Direction

- Preheat the oven to 375 Degrees F. Grease muffin pan or line with paper muffin liners.
- Mix together the flour, baking soda, baking powder and salt.
- In a separate bowl, beat together banana, sugar, egg, and vanilla (I used my kitchenaid.) Then add the dry ingredients to the wet ingredients and mix together until smooth and all ingredients are combined.
- Pour batter into prepared muffin tin, and bake for 15-18 minutes (or until toothpick comes out clean) Let cool completely before serving.
- ~Enjoy.

Nutrition Information

- Calories: 263.9
- Saturated Fat: 3.4
- Sodium: 407.6
- Total Carbohydrate: 49.9
- Total Fat: 6.4
- Fiber: 2.6
- Sugar: 23
- Cholesterol: 42.3
- Protein: 4.9

119. Double Apple Corn Muffins

Serving: 14 muffins, 14 serving(s) | Prep: 15mins | Ready in:

Ingredients

- 1 cup all-purpose flour
- 1 cup cornmeal
- 1/4 cup sugar
- 1 tablespoon baking powder
- 1/2 teaspoon salt
- 2 eggs, lightly beaten
- 2/3 cup unsweetened applesauce
- 1/2 cup milk
- 1/4 cup canola oil
- 1 large apple, peeled and finely chopped

Direction

- Stir together the flour, cornmeal, sugar, baking powder and salt; set aside.
- Combine the eggs, applesauce, milk and oil; stir into dry ingredients, just until moistened.
- Add apple.
- Spoon into greased muffin pans, filling 2/3 full.
- Bake at 425F for 15 minutes.
- Cool muffins five minutes in pan before serving.

Nutrition Information

- Calories: 141.7
- Total Fat: 5.3
- Sodium: 178.9
- Fiber: 1.4
- Sugar: 6.4
- Total Carbohydrate: 21.3
- Cholesterol: 27.8
- Saturated Fat: 0.8
- Protein: 2.9

120. Drop Biscuits

Serving: 12 serving(s) | Prep: 5mins | Ready in:

Ingredients

- 2 cups all-purpose flour
- 1 tablespoon baking powder
- 1 teaspoon sugar
- 1/4 cup chilled butter, , cut in small pieces
- 1 cup skim milk (or 1 or 2 %)

Direction

- The dough for these biscuits is dropped into muffin tins instead of onto a baking sheet, but their final shape is still like that of traditional drop biscuits.
- Preheat oven to 450 degrees.
- Lightly spoon flour into dry measuring cups, level with a knife.
- Combine flour, baking powder, sugar, and 1/2 teaspoon salt in a bowl, cut in butter with a pastry blender or 2 knives until mixture resembles coarse meal.
- Add milk, stir just until moist.
- Spoon batter in 12 muffin cups coated with cooking spray.
- Bake at 450 degrees for 12 minutes or until golden.
- Remove from pan immediately, place on a wire rack.
- Store any leftover biscuits in a zip loc plastic bag.
- To reheat in oven, wrap in foil.

Nutrition Information

- Calories: 120.1
- Sodium: 137.1
- Sugar: 0.4
- Protein: 3
- Total Fat: 4.1
- Fiber: 0.6
- Total Carbohydrate: 17.7
- Cholesterol: 10.6
- Saturated Fat: 2.5

121. Dutch Oven Breakfast Biscuits

Serving: 24 biscuits | Prep: 5mins | Ready in:

Ingredients

- 2 cups Bisquick
- 1 lb crumbled sausage
- 2/3 cup water, milk or 2/3 cup milk
- 1-2 cup shredded cheddar cheese

Direction

- Mix all together.
- Make large drop bisquits and place in oiled Dutch oven.
- Cook for about 20 minutes (depends on the number of briquettes used).
- Put on paper towels once removed to absorb excess grease.

Nutrition Information

- Calories: 122.2
- Saturated Fat: 3.2
- Sodium: 329.1
- Fiber: 0.2
- Sugar: 1.2
- Total Fat: 8.5
- Total Carbohydrate: 6.8
- Cholesterol: 16.1
- Protein: 4.2

122. Easiest Muffins By Trisha Yearwood

Serving: 12 muffins, 12 serving(s) | Prep: 5mins | Ready in:

Ingredients

- 1 cup margarine (softened)
- 1 cup sour cream
- 2 cups self-rising flour
- cooking spray

Direction

- Preheat the oven to 400 degrees F.
- In an electric mixer, cream the margarine and sour cream.
- Add the flour and mix well.

- Drop large spoonfuls of the dough into a muffin pan that has been sprayed with cooking spray or lined with muffin cups.
- Bake until the tops of the muffins are golden brown, 15 to 20 minutes.
- Cook's note: For smaller muffins, use mini muffin pans and reduce the baking time to 10 to 12 minutes.

Nutrition Information

- Calories: 178.4
- Total Fat: 11.6
- Protein: 2.5
- Saturated Fat: 3.8
- Sodium: 368.7
- Fiber: 0.6
- Sugar: 0.7
- Total Carbohydrate: 16.1
- Cholesterol: 10

123. Easiest Quickest (Low Cal) Pear (Any Fruit) Muffin For One

Serving: 1 serving(s) | Prep: 4mins | Ready in:

Ingredients

- 1 small pear, sliced
- 2 teaspoons cinnamon
- 1 g Splenda sugar substitute
- 2 tablespoons puffed rice cereal
- 1/2 egg white
- 1 teaspoon caramel syrup (optional)

Direction

- Slice fruit and microwave 25 secs.-check when tender.
- Spray muffin tin
- Preheat oven to 350.
- Mix egg, fruit, cinnamon, sugar, caramel.
- In separate cup mix cereal with a drop of water and loosely crush.
- Put egg mixture into muffin tin and top with cereal.
- Here you can add more sugar, cinnamon, and caramel--whatever you're feeling!
- Bake about 18 mins but check on it depending on your own preference (it should be crunchy on top and gooey and soft in the middle--sooooo good and low Cal I'd think too!

Nutrition Information

- Calories: 111.4
- Total Fat: 0.3
- Sodium: 30
- Fiber: 6.8
- Sugar: 14.6
- Cholesterol: 0
- Saturated Fat: 0
- Total Carbohydrate: 27.7
- Protein: 2.6

124. Easy Banana Choc Chip Mini Muffins

Serving: 36 serving(s) | Prep: 5mins | Ready in:

Ingredients

- 500 g vanilla cake mix
- 2 eggs
- 1/3 cup olive oil
- 3 bananas, mashed
- 1/2 cup chocolate chips

Direction

- Preheat 180 C in fan forced oven.
- Heat peeled bananas in the microwave until soft and mash with a fork, allow to cool.
- Mix together oil and eggs in a bowl with a whisk and add mashed banana, combine well.

- Add cake mix and choc chips and mix until just combine with a wooden spoon.
- Spray a mini muffin tray with canola oil spray.
- Bake for 20 to 25 minute.

Nutrition Information

- Calories: 101.7
- Sodium: 95.5
- Fiber: 0.6
- Sugar: 8.5
- Protein: 1.2
- Total Fat: 4.6
- Saturated Fat: 1
- Total Carbohydrate: 14.6
- Cholesterol: 12

125. Easy Blue Cheese Biscuits

Serving: 32-40 mini biscuits | Prep: 10mins | Ready in:

Ingredients

- 1/2 cup butter
- 2 -3 ounces blue cheese, crumbled
- 1 (8 -10 count) can refrigerated biscuits

Direction

- Preheat oven to 375 degrees. Blend crumbled blue cheese and melted butter in a bowl.
- Cut each biscuit into fourths and dip each into butter mixture.
- Place on baking sheet or in mini muffin pans and bake for about 12-15 minutes. Serve warm.

Nutrition Information

- Calories: 55.2
- Sodium: 126.3
- Sugar: 0.6
- Total Fat: 4.4

- Saturated Fat: 2.4
- Total Carbohydrate: 3.2
- Cholesterol: 8.9
- Protein: 0.9
- Fiber: 0.1

126. Easy Cheese Muffins

Serving: 12 muffins | Prep: 10mins | Ready in:

Ingredients

- 2 cups flour, unsifted
- 3 teaspoons baking powder
- 1/2 cup mayonnaise, Hellman's works just fine
- 1 cup milk
- 1 1/2 cups grated cheese

Direction

- Mix together dry ingredients and mayonnaise, then add milk and mix.
- Add the grated cheese and mix.
- Grease a 12 muffin pan and divide dough equally between.
- Bake in a preheated 450 degree F oven for 20 minutes.

Nutrition Information

- Calories: 174.4
- Total Fat: 7.7
- Saturated Fat: 3.1
- Sodium: 307.2
- Fiber: 0.6
- Total Carbohydrate: 20.6
- Cholesterol: 14.4
- Sugar: 0.7
- Protein: 5.7

127. Easy English Scones

Serving: 18 scones, 6-8 serving(s) | Prep: 10mins | Ready in:

Ingredients

- 2 cups sifted all-purpose flour (256gm)
- 1/2 cup white sugar
- 2 1/2 teaspoons baking powder
- 1/2 teaspoon baking soda
- 1/2 teaspoon salt (3ml)
- 1/4 cup margarine (I use 5 tbsp on a butter stick) or 1/4 cup butter (I use 5 tbsp on a butter stick)
- 3/4 cup sultana raisin (in a pinch regular raisins will do fine)
- 1 cup milk
- 1/2 cup sweetened flaked coconut

Direction

- Preheat oven to 425°F or 220°C and grease baking tray with margarine ready.
- Sift the flour, sugar, baking powder, baking soda and salt together.
- Cut in the margarine or butter till mixture resembles very fine breadcrumbs, then stir in the raisins and coconut.
- Add the milk and mix to make a smooth dough. (Adding a little more milk if necessary. The mix should not be too dry).
- Knead very lightly for ten seconds on a lightly floured surface. Roll or pat to about 3/4" thick (2 cm) and either cut into individual scones.
- Bake for approximately 12 minutes (makes about 18 scones).

Nutrition Information

- Calories: 370.1
- Saturated Fat: 4.2
- Fiber: 2.1
- Total Carbohydrate: 68.9
- Protein: 6.5
- Total Fat: 8.5
- Sodium: 537.6
- Sugar: 30.8
- Cholesterol: 5.7

128. Easy French Onion Biscuits

Serving: 6-12 Biscuits, 6-12 serving(s) | Prep: 5mins | Ready in:

Ingredients

- 2 cups Bisquick
- 1/4 cup milk
- 1 (8 ounce) container French onion dip
- 1/2 cup white cheddar cheese, grated
- 1/2 teaspoon dried parsley
- 1/2 teaspoon paprika

Direction

- Biscuits -- Mix the Bisquick, milk onion dip, parsley.
- Bake -- Just drop spoonfuls of the mix on a baking sheet lined with parchment paper or sprayed with a non-stick spray. Top with the grated cheese and a light sprinkle of the paprika.
- Bake at 400 degrees until golden brown. 12-18 minutes. Just check, because all pans, biscuit size and ovens vary. You just want them golden brown. ENJOY! Don't forget to serve with an herb butter. I can buy a stick of herb butter right at my grocery store. Makes a nice touch to the biscuits.

Nutrition Information

- Calories: 222.6
- Fiber: 0.9
- Sugar: 4.7
- Protein: 6.3
- Total Fat: 10.2
- Sodium: 583.9
- Total Carbohydrate: 26

- Cholesterol: 13.8
- Saturated Fat: 4.1

129. Easy Herb Biscuits

Serving: 12 serving(s) | Prep: 5mins | Ready in:

Ingredients

- cooking spray
- 2 cups self-rising flour
- 1 1/2 teaspoons fresh sage, chopped (or favorite herb) or 1/4 teaspoon dried sage
- 1 1/2 teaspoons fresh thyme, chopped (or favorite herb) or 1/4 teaspoon dried thyme
- 1/4 cup mayonnaise
- 1 cup milk (or buttermilk)

Direction

- Preheat oven to 400*F. Spray nonstick a nonstick 12-cup muffin pan with vegetable oil.
- Whisk sage and thyme into the flour.
- Using a large dinner fork, stir in the mayonnaise and milk (or buttermilk) until combined. Do not over mix.
- Divide batter evenly into muffin cups.
- Bake in preheated oven for 12 to 15 minutes until golden.
- My Note: Do not mix up the biscuits too far in advance in order to retain the action of the leavening powder. This recipe is particularly good with poultry and pork. Feel free to vary the herbs to your tastes. The batter is also great as a topping for pot pies in place of a rolled crust.
- This was amazing from beginning to eating. I had guests for dinner the first time I tried it. I doubled the batch, opted for butter milk, and used fresh herbs from my wife's garden. I served the biscuits with homemade spaghetti instead of the normal garlic or French bread. I went really well. One of my guests does not cook. After watching me make it, she remarked "Even I could make that." At the end of the evening, she asked to take the left over biscuits home, and asked for the recipe. She attends a church that has monthly potluck lunches. She says now she can bring something to the potluck that does not come pre made from the store.
- In my oven, I had to cook them for 17 minutes to get a nice brown. I would not hesitate to serve this to guest, or even enter it into competition (county fair, etc.) and have the confidence they would do very well. I am looking forward to using them with my all-time favorite, good 'ol biscuits and gravy.

Nutrition Information

- Calories: 106.2
- Protein: 2.8
- Fiber: 0.6
- Sugar: 0.4
- Cholesterol: 4.1
- Total Fat: 2.6
- Saturated Fat: 0.7
- Sodium: 309.4
- Total Carbohydrate: 17.7

130. Easy Low Fat Cornbread

Serving: 12 serving(s) | Prep: 10mins | Ready in:

Ingredients

- 1 1/4 cups flour
- 3/4 cup cornmeal
- 1/4 cup sugar
- 2 teaspoons baking powder
- 1/4 teaspoon baking soda
- 1/2 teaspoon salt
- 1 1/4 cups low-fat buttermilk (slightly more if too thick)
- 1 egg

Direction

- Combine dry ingredients in mixing bowl.
- Add egg and buttermilk and blend well.
- Spread into an 8x8 baking dish sprayed with vegetable spray or spoon into prepared muffin tins and bake in a 400 degree oven for 20-25 minutes or until toothpick inserted near center comes out clean.

Nutrition Information

- Calories: 107.8
- Sodium: 219.2
- Fiber: 0.9
- Sugar: 5.5
- Cholesterol: 18.6
- Saturated Fat: 0.3
- Total Carbohydrate: 21.4
- Protein: 3.3
- Total Fat: 1

131. Easy Sourdough Biscuits(Bisquick)

Serving: 10 biscuits, 5 serving(s) | Prep: 5mins | Ready in:

Ingredients

- 1 cup sourdough starter
- 1 cup Bisquick (I used homemade)

Direction

- Mix together.
- Knead gently on a lightly floured surface.
- Roll to about 1/2 to 3/4 inch thick and cut out biscuits (I use a jelly jar glass).
- Place on ungreased cookie sheet.
- Bake at 400°F for 12 to 15 minutes.

Nutrition Information

- Calories: 109.6
- Saturated Fat: 1

- Sodium: 259.1
- Fiber: 0.5
- Cholesterol: 0.5
- Protein: 2
- Total Fat: 3.9
- Sugar: 3
- Total Carbohydrate: 16.2

132. Eating Suburbia's Banana Oatmeal Scones

Serving: 16 scones, 8 serving(s) | Prep: 15mins | Ready in:

Ingredients

- 2 cups all-purpose flour
- 1/4 cup sugar
- 1 tablespoon baking powder
- 1 teaspoon cream of tartar
- 1/2 teaspoon salt
- 1 1/4 cups old-fashioned oatmeal (1 minute oats can be used)
- 1/2 cup margarine or 1/2 cup butter, melted
- 1/3 cup soya milk, plain or 1/3 cup soya milk, vanilla or 1/3 cup milk
- 1 banana, ripe mashed
- Optional additions
- 1/4-1/2 cup chocolate chips or 1/4-1/2 cup walnuts or 1/4-1/2 cup pecans or 1 tablespoon crystalyzed ginger

Direction

- Combine dry ingredients; set aside.
- Blend mashed banana, melted margarine, and soy milk until fairly smooth. Add in dry ingredients and optional item and mix just until moistened. Pour out onto floured board. Incorporate more flour if dough is too sticky. Cut dough in half and roll or pat each half into a circle, about 7-8 inches around. Cut into 8 wedges. Place on silpat or oiled baking sheet.
- Bake 425 for about 10 minutes, until light golden brown.

Nutrition Information

- Calories: 282.2
- Sodium: 355.5
- Total Carbohydrate: 46.7
- Cholesterol: 0
- Total Fat: 8.6
- Saturated Fat: 2.3
- Fiber: 2.9
- Sugar: 11.5
- Protein: 5.7

133. Elderberry Muffins

Serving: 12 muffins | Prep: 10mins | Ready in:

Ingredients

- 1 cup sugar
- 1/2 cup oleo
- 1 cup milk
- 1 egg
- 1 teaspoon nutmeg
- 1 1/2 cups flour
- 1/8 teaspoon salt
- 2 teaspoons baking powder
- 1/2 teaspoon cinnamon
- 3/4 cup wheat germ
- 3 tablespoons molasses
- 1/2 cup dried elderberries

Direction

- Cream sugar and oleo, add additional ingredients and mix until blended.
- Bake at 425 degrees for 20 minutes in a muffin pan.

Nutrition Information

- Calories: 250.1
- Total Carbohydrate: 37.5
- Cholesterol: 20.5
- Protein: 4.6
- Sodium: 192.3
- Fiber: 1.5
- Sugar: 19.6
- Total Fat: 9.7
- Saturated Fat: 2.2

134. Even Healthier Morning Glory Muffins

Serving: 12 muffins | Prep: 10mins | Ready in:

Ingredients

- 1 cup all-purpose flour
- 1 cup whole wheat flour
- 3/4 cup ground flax seeds
- 3/4 cup brown sugar
- 2 3/4 teaspoons baking powder
- 2 teaspoons ground cinnamon
- 1/2 teaspoon nutmeg
- 1/4 teaspoon salt
- 1 1/2 teaspoons baking soda
- 4 egg whites
- 1 egg
- 1/2 cup unsweetened applesauce
- 7 ounces crushed pineapple, reserve juice
- 2 teaspoons vanilla extract
- 2 cups carrots, grated
- 1/2 cup raisins

Direction

- In a large bowl, combine the Dry ingredients.
- In another bowl, beat the egg whites and egg, add other wet ingredients. Mix together - if too dry add pineapple juice - if too wet add more all-purpose flour (a bit at a time) time.
- Use muffin liners; fill three-fourths full. Bake at 350 degrees F for 15-18 minutes or until a toothpick comes out clean. Cool for 5 minutes before removing from pans to wire.

Nutrition Information

- Calories: 216.8
- Sugar: 20.4
- Total Carbohydrate: 41.7
- Cholesterol: 17.6
- Sodium: 335.1
- Fiber: 4.6
- Saturated Fat: 0.5
- Protein: 5.9
- Total Fat: 3.8

135. Fat Free Banana Bread

Serving: 1 Loaf, or dozen + mini muffins, 1 serving(s) | Prep: 10mins | Ready in:

Ingredients

- 3 mashed bananas (ripe, with brown spots makes them sweeter!)
- 1 1/2 cups Splenda sugar substitute
- 1/2 cup applesauce
- 2 eggs, whites** (I used the boxed or fridge kind)
- 1/4 cup almond milk
- 1 1/2 cups whole wheat flour
- 1 teaspoon baking soda
- 1/2 cup gluten free chocolate chips (or more) (optional)

Direction

- Mix together in order. Pour into lightly palmed 9*5" loaf pan. Bake at 350°F for 1 hour 20 minutes. Or In a muffin tin for 40 minutes. Let cool and ENJOY!
- **I edited this recipe as it originally came out as 15g fat and over 2000 cals. Splenda, egg whites, and bananas do not add to over 2k cals! Silly Recipezaar calorie calculator :-).
- *VEGAN TIP: You can easily make this bread VEGAN by mixing 2 tablespoons ground flax seed (or flax meal) with 6 tablespoons of hot water. Use this mixture in replace of the eggs!

Nutrition Information

- Calories: 1169.2
- Sodium: 1446.8
- Fiber: 32.7
- Sugar: 44.8
- Total Carbohydrate: 237.6
- Cholesterol: 423
- Protein: 41.3
- Total Fat: 14.7
- Saturated Fat: 4.1

136. Fat Free Cranberry Orange Muffins

Serving: 12 muffins | Prep: 5mins | Ready in:

Ingredients

- 2 cups all-purpose flour
- 1 teaspoon baking powder
- 1/2 teaspoon baking soda
- 1/2 teaspoon salt
- 1/2 cup sugar
- 2 egg whites
- 1/4 cup unsweetened applesauce
- 2/3 cup orange juice
- 2 teaspoons grated orange zest
- 2/3 cup craisins

Direction

- Whisk together the dry, then the wet. Gradually whisk in the dry to the wet. Fold in cranberries and bake 16-18 minutes at 400, make sure you grease the cups!

Nutrition Information

- Calories: 140.4
- Cholesterol: 0
- Protein: 2.9
- Total Fat: 0.3
- Saturated Fat: 0

- Fiber: 1.1
- Total Carbohydrate: 31.9
- Sodium: 189.6
- Sugar: 13.9

137. Fat Free, Sugar Free Cholesterol Free Blueberry Muffins!

Serving: 8 serving(s) | Prep: 10mins | Ready in:

Ingredients

- 1 cup unsweetened blueberries (fresh or frozen)
- 1 3/4 cups all-purpose flour (I use the "unbleached" kind)
- 2 1/2 teaspoons baking powder
- 1/3 cup Splenda granular
- 1/4 cup Egg Beaters egg substitute (equals 1 egg)
- 1/4 cup unsweetened applesauce
- 1/2 cup nonfat milk (skim)
- 1 tablespoon Splenda granular (to top muffins)

Direction

- Preheat oven to 400 degrees.
- Lightly spray muffin tin with non-stick spray (I've found that paper muffin holders do not peel away from these muffins easily).
- Wash and drain blueberries. Set aside. If using frozen blueberries, thaw before using.
- In large bowl, sift flour. Add baking powder and the 1/3 cup Splenda. Mix together.
- In another bowl, mix the Egg Beater egg substitute, apple sauce and milk.
- Combine the wet mixture into the flour mixture. Stir just enough to blend (electric mixers aren't really necessary). Gently fold in the blueberries.
- Pour batter into the prepared muffin tin, filling each cup about 2/3 full. Use the last tablespoon of Splenda to sprinkle on top of each muffin (this adds zero calories and has zero fat) and bake for 17 minutes, or until tops are light brown.
- After baking, allow muffins to cool before removing them from the tin. Please note: 1 serving = 1 muffin. Enjoy!

Nutrition Information

- Calories: 118.5
- Saturated Fat: 0.1
- Sodium: 120.8
- Protein: 3.4
- Total Fat: 0.4
- Fiber: 1.4
- Sugar: 3.2
- Total Carbohydrate: 25.2
- Cholesterol: 0.3

138. Fiber Rich Muffins

Serving: 12 serving(s) | Prep: 10mins | Ready in:

Ingredients

- 1 cup multi-grain hot cereal
- 1 cup unbleached white flour
- 1 tablespoon baking powder
- 1/2 teaspoon baking soda
- 1/2 teaspoon salt
- 1/2 cup sugar
- 1 cup carrot, shredded
- 1 cup apple, peeled chopped
- 1/2 cup milk
- 2 eggs or 4 egg whites
- 1/4 cup vegetable oil
- 1 teaspoon vanilla
- 1/2 cup pecans, chopped

Direction

- Preheat oven to 400*F.
- Line 12 muffin cups with paper liners or grease muffin cups.

- Blend together dry ingredients. Add remaining ingredients and mix until blended.
- Batter will be thick; spoon into muffin cups. Bake 20-22 minutes or until golden brown.

Nutrition Information

- Calories: 171.2
- Protein: 3
- Total Fat: 9.2
- Sugar: 10.1
- Total Carbohydrate: 20.1
- Cholesterol: 36.7
- Saturated Fat: 1.4
- Sodium: 263.4
- Fiber: 1.2

139. French Toast Scones

Serving: 12 serving(s) | Prep: 15mins | Ready in:

Ingredients

- 2 cups flour (can use half all purpose and half pastry flour, thats what I do)
- 4 teaspoons baking powder
- 1/2 teaspoon salt
- 1/3 cup sugar
- 4 tablespoons butter
- 2/3 cup milk
- 1 egg
- 1/2 teaspoon butter flavoring
- 1/2 teaspoon maple flavoring
- 4 1/2 tablespoons maple syrup
- 1/3 cup cinnamon baking chips (you can add more if you like)

Direction

- Mix the flour, baking powder, salt, and sugar together.
- Cut in the butter. A food processor works best, but doing by hand will work too. Just make sure there is no chunks of butter left over after cutting into mixture. And then put the flour mixture in a large bowl. Mix cinnamon chips into the flour mixture.
- Whisk together the milk, egg, butter flavoring, maple flavoring, and maple syrup in separate bowl then add to flour mixture, mix together.
- If the mixture is to thin add a little flour till it is a consistency you can work with. Take out of bowl and make into a ball, flatten to where it is about an inch thick. Cut into about 12 or less pie type slices (Depends how big you want them) and put onto a lightly greased cookie sheet.
- Cook at 450 for 12-15 minutes.

Nutrition Information

- Calories: 166.6
- Protein: 3.2
- Saturated Fat: 2.9
- Total Carbohydrate: 27.5
- Sugar: 10.2
- Cholesterol: 27.6
- Total Fat: 4.9
- Sodium: 265.7
- Fiber: 0.6

140. Fresh Tomato Biscuits

Serving: 10 biscuits | Prep: 5mins | Ready in:

Ingredients

- 1/4 cup mayonnaise
- 1/4 teaspoon salt
- 1/4 teaspoon fresh coarse ground black pepper
- 1/4 cup shredded fresh basil
- 1 (16 1/3 ounce) can ready-to-bake refrigerated buttermilk flaky biscuits
- 2 medium tomatoes, thinly sliced

Direction

- Combine first 4 ingredients. Set aside.

- Press each biscuit into a 4-inch circle. Place biscuit circles on a lightly greased baking sheet.
- Bake at 400° for 6 minutes. Spread each biscuit evenly with about 2 teaspoons mayonnaise mixture. Top evenly with tomato slices. Bake at 400° for 6 more minutes or until mayonnaise mixture is bubbly. Serve immediately.

Nutrition Information

- Calories: 150.2
- Sodium: 413.2
- Cholesterol: 1.5
- Protein: 3.1
- Total Fat: 4.6
- Saturated Fat: 0.9
- Fiber: 0.3
- Sugar: 1
- Total Carbohydrate: 24.5

141. Fried Hot Water Cornbread

Serving: 6-8 patties, 4 serving(s) | Prep: 15mins | Ready in:

Ingredients

- 1 cup self-rising cornmeal
- 1/3 cup self-rising flour
- 1 cup boiling water
- oil (for frying)

Direction

- Mix cornmeal and flour in mixing bowl.
- Pour in boiling water (may need to add a little more to make mixture stick together.
- Stir well.
- Let cool for a few minutes.
- Preheat iron skillet or griddle and add enough oil to cover bottom of skillet.
- Spoon about 1/4 cup into hot skillet.
- Brown on both sides.
- Drain on paper towel and serve while still hot.

Nutrition Information

- Calories: 138.7
- Saturated Fat: 0.2
- Fiber: 2.3
- Sugar: 0
- Cholesterol: 0
- Protein: 3.5
- Total Fat: 1.1
- Sodium: 514.3
- Total Carbohydrate: 29.2

142. Fruit Filled Muffins

Serving: 12 serving(s) | Prep: 10mins | Ready in:

Ingredients

- 2/3 cup milk
- 1 tablespoon vegetable oil
- 1 egg
- 2 cups original Bisquick baking mix
- 1/4 cup fruit preserves (any flavor)
- 2/3 cup powdered sugar
- Icing
- 2/3 cup powdered sugar
- 4 teaspoons water

Direction

- Heat oven to 400°F
- Grease bottoms only of 12 regular-size muffin cups with shortening or cooking spray, or line with paper baking cups.
- Stir milk, oil and egg until blended.
- Stir in Bisquick mix and sugar.
- Divide batter evenly among muffin cups. Drop 1 level teaspoon fruit preserves onto center of batter in each cup.
- Bake 13 to 18 minutes or until golden brown.

- Mix powdered sugar and water until smooth. Allow muffins to cool slightly before drizzling icing over warm muffins.

Nutrition Information

- Calories: 180.8
- Total Fat: 5.1
- Sugar: 18.7
- Protein: 2.6
- Saturated Fat: 1.4
- Sodium: 270
- Fiber: 0.5
- Total Carbohydrate: 31.2
- Cholesterol: 19.9

143. Gem Scones

Serving: 12 scones | Prep: 10mins | Ready in:

Ingredients

- 1 1/4 cups self raising flour
- 2 tablespoons butter, level
- 1 egg
- 155 ml milk
- 3 tablespoons sugar, level
- 1/2 teaspoon salt

Direction

- Preheat oven to 200 degrees C (400 degrees F).
- Heat gem irons.
- Cream butter and sugar; add egg, beat well then add milk.
- Lastly add sifted flour and mix in lightly.
- Spoon into heated, greased gem irons.
- Cook 7 to 10 minutes.
- Best served warm with butter.

Nutrition Information

- Calories: 90.8
- Sodium: 122.8
- Fiber: 0.3
- Protein: 2.3
- Total Carbohydrate: 13.7
- Cholesterol: 24.5
- Total Fat: 2.9
- Saturated Fat: 1.6
- Sugar: 3.2

144. Ginger Molasses Muffins

Serving: 12 medium muffins | Prep: 5mins | Ready in:

Ingredients

- 2 1/2 cups all-purpose flour, unbleached
- 1/2 cup light brown sugar, packed
- 1 tablespoon ground ginger
- 2 teaspoons baking powder
- 1 teaspoon baking soda
- 1/2 teaspoon ground cloves
- 1 cup buttermilk
- 1/2 cup dark molasses, unsulphured
- 1/4 cup vegetable oil
- 1 large egg

Direction

- Preheat oven to 400* --
- Lightly grease, spray or line 12 muffin cups with paper liners and set aside.
- Combine flour, brown sugar, ginger, baking powder, baking soda, and cloves in a large bowl, and stir till well blended.
- In a separate bowl, whisk together the buttermilk, molasses, oil and egg.
- Add to the dry ingredients all at once and fold just until the dry ingredients are evenly moistened.
- Do not overmix.
- Divide the batter evenly among the muffin cups.
- Bake until the edges begin to pull away from sides and a toothpick inserted in the centers comes out clean -- 20-22 minutes.
- Cool on wire rack before removing from pans.

Nutrition Information

- Calories: 226.8
- Protein: 4
- Saturated Fat: 0.9
- Sodium: 201.4
- Sugar: 17.8
- Total Carbohydrate: 40.9
- Total Fat: 5.4
- Fiber: 0.8
- Cholesterol: 16.3

145. Gingernut Biscuits

Serving: 60 cookies | Prep: 15mins | Ready in:

Ingredients

- 200 g butter (7 oz)
- 1 cup sugar
- 1 cup golden syrup
- 3 cups flour
- 1 tablespoon ground ginger (heaped)
- 1 teaspoon baking soda

Direction

- Pre heat oven to 350°F (180°C).
- Cream the butter and the sugar.
- Add the golden syrup and the dry ingredients.
- Mix everything together and roll into little balls. Put onto a greased baking tray, pressing the balls down very slightly with a fork.
- Bake at 350°F and 180°C for 15 minutes.
- Cool on a wire rack and keep in an airtight container once cold.

Nutrition Information

- Calories: 75.8
- Saturated Fat: 1.7
- Sodium: 48.3
- Sugar: 4.9
- Total Carbohydrate: 12.5
- Protein: 0.7
- Total Fat: 2.8
- Fiber: 0.2
- Cholesterol: 7.1

146. Glazed Blueberry Biscuits

Serving: 10 biscuits, 10 serving(s) | Prep: 15mins | Ready in:

Ingredients

- 2 cups flour
- 1/3 cup sugar
- 4 teaspoons baking powder
- 1 teaspoon salt
- 1 cup milk, cold
- 5 tablespoons butter, frozen
- 3 ounces blueberries (fresh or dried)
- 1 tablespoon butter, melted
- 1 cup powdered sugar
- 2 tablespoons water
- 1 teaspoon vanilla
- 1/2 teaspoon lemon juice

Direction

- Preheat oven to 450°F.
- Whisk flour, sugar, baking powder and salt in a large bowl until well-incorporated.
- Add the cold milk mix a bit. As dough begins to form, use a cheese grater to grate the butter into the dough evenly. Fold dough as you grate so the butter spreads evenly throughout. When done with the butter, fold in the blueberries.
- Gently pull off chunks of dough and pat to form 10 biscuits of roughly the same size. Place on ungreased cookie sheet or cake pan. Bake in oven for about 7-12 minutes, or until golden.
- When biscuits are done, paint them with the melted butter using a pastry brush.

- Just before serving, mix the powdered sugar, water, vanilla and lemon juice to create a glaze. Drizzle over biscuits.

Nutrition Information

- Calories: 247.3
- Sodium: 451.6
- Fiber: 0.9
- Sugar: 19.4
- Total Fat: 8.1
- Saturated Fat: 5
- Total Carbohydrate: 40.6
- Cholesterol: 21.7
- Protein: 3.5

147. Gluten Free Casein Free Applesauce Muffins

Serving: 12 muffins, 4 serving(s) | Prep: 10mins | Ready in:

Ingredients

- 1 cup rice flour
- 1/2 cup cornstarch
- 1/2 cup sugar
- 1 1/2 teaspoons cinnamon
- 1 teaspoon salt
- 1 teaspoon baking soda
- 3/4 teaspoon guar gum
- 1 cup applesauce
- 1/2 cup canola oil
- 1/4 cup rice milk
- 1 egg

Direction

- Preheat oven to 400 degrees Fahrenheit and line 12-cup muffin pan with paper liners.
- Combine all ingredients in large mixing bowl; mix just until blended.
- Divide muffin batter evenly in prepared pan.

- Bake for 12-18 minutes or until toothpick inserted in center of one muffin comes out clean.

Nutrition Information

- Calories: 611.9
- Total Fat: 29.1
- Sodium: 933.4
- Sugar: 25.1
- Total Carbohydrate: 84.8
- Protein: 4.1
- Saturated Fat: 2.6
- Fiber: 2.4
- Cholesterol: 46.5

148. Good Morning Muffins

Serving: 12 muffins | Prep: 10mins | Ready in:

Ingredients

- Dry Ingredients
- 1 1/2 cups flour
- 1 teaspoon baking powder
- 1 teaspoon baking soda
- 1/2 teaspoon salt
- 1/2 teaspoon cinnamon
- 1/4 teaspoon nutmeg
- 1/8 teaspoon ginger
- 1/8 teaspoon allspice
- 3/4 cup brown sugar
- Wet Ingredients
- 1 egg
- 1/2 cup yogurt
- 1/4 cup oil
- 1/2 teaspoon vanilla
- 1 (7 ounce) canUndrained crushed pineapple
- 3/4 cup grated carrot
- 1/2 cup raisins

Direction

- Preheat oven to 400.

- Combine dry ingredients in a large bowl.
- Beat together wet ingredients and pour into dry mixture.
- Stir just until combined.
- Fill muffin cups and bake for 15- 17 minutes.

Nutrition Information

- Calories: 193.3
- Saturated Fat: 1
- Sodium: 253.9
- Sugar: 20.1
- Protein: 2.8
- Total Fat: 5.5
- Fiber: 1
- Total Carbohydrate: 34.1
- Cholesterol: 18.9

149. Grandma's Best Scones

Serving: 12 scones | Prep: 10mins | Ready in:

Ingredients

- 45 g butter
- 1 1/2 tablespoons sugar
- 1 egg
- 1 pinch salt
- 2 cups self-raising flour
- 1/2 cup milk
- 1/2 cup sultana

Direction

- Cream butter and sugar until light and fluffy.
- Add beaten egg and salt.
- Add sifted flour and milk alternately, mix to a soft dough, add sultanas.
- Turn on to lightly-floured surface, knead slightly.
- Roll out to 2 cm thickness, cut with round scone cutter.
- Put scones on greased oven tray, bake in hot oven (230 C) 7 to 10 minutes.

Nutrition Information

- Calories: 140
- Sugar: 5.7
- Protein: 3.2
- Fiber: 0.8
- Sodium: 310.6
- Total Carbohydrate: 23
- Cholesterol: 27.1
- Total Fat: 4
- Saturated Fat: 2.3

150. Great Biscuits

Serving: 20-22 serving(s) | Prep: 10mins | Ready in:

Ingredients

- 1 cup self rising flour
- 1/2 cup butter or 1/2 cup margarine (set it out for 8-10 minutes or so)
- 1/2 cup sour cream

Direction

- Mix the ingredients together.
- Roll the dough and cut the biscuits about 1/2 inch thick.
- Bake at 400 degrees for 10-15 minutes (oven variation). I use a cast iron biscuit skillet.

Nutrition Information

- Calories: 75.1
- Saturated Fat: 3.7
- Sodium: 115.1
- Sugar: 0
- Total Carbohydrate: 4.9
- Cholesterol: 14.7
- Total Fat: 5.9
- Fiber: 0.2
- Protein: 0.8

151. Grilled Egg Cheese And Bacon Biscuit

Serving: 4 serving(s) | Prep: 10mins | Ready in:

Ingredients

- 4 large eggs, beaten
- 1 tablespoon milk
- 1/4 teaspoon salt
- 1/4 teaspoon pepper
- 6 tablespoons butter, divided
- 4 biscuits, halved
- 4 slices bacon, cooked
- 1/4 cup shredded cheddar cheese

Direction

- In bowl, combine eggs, milk, salt and pepper.
- In skillet melt 1 tablespoon butter over medium heat. Cook eggs. Set aside and wipe skillet clean.
- Spread remaining butter over biscuits. Top with eggs, bacon and cheese. Replace tops. Fry in skillet until cheese is melted and biscuits are lightly browned.

Nutrition Information

- Calories: 503.9
- Total Carbohydrate: 27.6
- Cholesterol: 247
- Protein: 13.5
- Total Fat: 37.9
- Saturated Fat: 17.9
- Sodium: 828.8
- Fiber: 0.9
- Sugar: 1.5

152. Ham Pineapple Pizza Muffins

Serving: 8 serving(s) | Prep: 10mins | Ready in:

Ingredients

- 4 English muffins
- 1/2 cup tomato paste
- 1 teaspoon dried oregano
- 440 g pineapple chunks in juice, drained
- 150 g ham, chopped
- 200 g grated mozzarella cheese

Direction

- Split each muffin in half, spread each with the paste, and top each muffin with the pineapple, ham then cheese and oregano. Place muffins on oven tray in moderate oven for about 15 - 20 minutes, or until cheese is melted and pizzas are heated through.
- Serve immediately.

Nutrition Information

- Calories: 214.1
- Cholesterol: 29.5
- Protein: 13.2
- Saturated Fat: 3.9
- Sodium: 674.6
- Fiber: 2.2
- Sugar: 11.2
- Total Carbohydrate: 25
- Total Fat: 7.3

153. Ham Or Sausage Cheese Muffins

Serving: 12 serving(s) | Prep: 10mins | Ready in:

Ingredients

- 2 cups self rising flour

- 1 teaspoon baking soda
- 1 cup milk
- 1/2 cup mayonnaise
- 1/2 cup fully cooked chopped ham or 1/2 cup sausage (drain grease if using sausage)
- 1/2 cup sharp shredded cheddar cheese

Direction

- In a large bowl combine flour, baking soda.
- Combine remaining ingredients.
- Stir into dry ingredients just until moistened.
- Fill greased or paper lined muffin cups 2/3 full.
- Bake at 425 degrees for 14 minutes or until muffins test done.

Nutrition Information

- Calories: 152.5
- Protein: 5.3
- Fiber: 0.6
- Total Carbohydrate: 18.8
- Cholesterol: 13.4
- Sodium: 566.7
- Sugar: 0.7
- Total Fat: 6.1
- Saturated Fat: 2.1

154. Healthy Apricot Walnut Muffins

Serving: 12 serving(s) | Prep: 10mins | Ready in:

Ingredients

- 1 1/2 cups white whole wheat flour or 1 1/2 cups white bread flour
- 3/4 cup uncooked oatmeal, any kind
- 1/2 cup wheat germ or 1/2 cup another 1/2 cup flour
- 1/2 cup brown sugar
- 2 teaspoons baking powder
- 1/2 teaspoon baking soda
- 1/4 teaspoon salt
- 1 teaspoon cinnamon
- 2 eggs, lightly beaten
- 3/4 cup buttermilk or 3/4 cup milk
- 3 tablespoons melted butter
- 1/2 cup chopped dried apricot
- 1/2 cup chopped walnuts

Direction

- In large bowl mix together flour, oatmeal, wheat germ, brown sugar, baking soda, baking powder, salt, cinnamon, and mix all well together.
- Add eggs, buttermilk, mix in flour mixture. Next add melted butter and mix well. Line muffin pan with liners or spray with nonstick spray. Divide muffin batter evenly between 12 muffin liners. Top each muffin with chopped walnuts and lightly sprinkle with additional cinnamon and granulated sugar over each.
- Bake muffins in 375 degrees preheated oven for 20 minutes. Test muffins for doneness with a toothpick, set toothpick in middle of muffin and if the tooth pick comes out clean the muffins are done, otherwise bake a couple additional minutes and test again. To see additional photos of Healthy Apricot Walnut Muffins and other recipes see sliceoftaste.com.

Nutrition Information

- Calories: 211.6
- Cholesterol: 39.2
- Saturated Fat: 2.7
- Sodium: 219.1
- Fiber: 3.6
- Sugar: 12.8
- Total Carbohydrate: 30.9
- Total Fat: 8.2
- Protein: 6.3

155. Healthy Banana Muffins

Serving: 16 muffins | Prep: 15mins | Ready in:

Ingredients

- 1/2 cup oat bran
- 1/2 cup kamut flour
- 1/4 cup brown rice flour
- 1 cup whole wheat flour
- 1 teaspoon baking soda
- 1 1/2 teaspoons baking powder
- 1 teaspoon cinnamon
- 1/2 teaspoon salt
- 1/2 cup brown sugar
- 1/4 cup flax seed
- 1 teaspoon vanilla extract
- 1/2 teaspoon almond extract
- 4 egg whites
- 1/2 cup vanilla-flavored soymilk
- 2 cups mashed bananas
- 1/4 cup olive oil

Direction

- Mix all dry ingredients together.
- Mix remaining ingredients.
- Combine all ingredients, mix until completely moist.
- Preheat oven 400 degrees.
- Bake for 20 minutes in a muffin tin coated with cooking spray.

Nutrition Information

- Calories: 134.1
- Total Fat: 5
- Sugar: 9.2
- Total Carbohydrate: 21.3
- Saturated Fat: 0.7
- Sodium: 203.6
- Fiber: 2.8
- Cholesterol: 0
- Protein: 3.3

156. Healthy Banana Nut Muffins

Serving: 12 muffins | Prep: 10mins | Ready in:

Ingredients

- 1/2 cup oat bran
- 1/2 cup whole wheat flour
- 1/4 cup brown sugar
- 1 cup soymilk lite
- 1/4 cup egg white
- 1 tablespoon canola oil
- 2 teaspoons baking powder
- 2 teaspoons baking soda
- 1 banana
- 1 teaspoon vanilla extract
- 1/4 cup walnuts

Direction

- Preheat oven to 430 degrees.
- Pour all ingredients into a bowl, and mix thoroughly (sometimes it helps to mash the banana in a separate container before adding to bowl). Also, if you prefer your muffins sweeter, add around 5 or 6 artificial sweetener packets to the batter.
- Cook for around 10 minutes.

Nutrition Information

- Calories: 82.9
- Cholesterol: 0
- Sugar: 5.8
- Sodium: 281.1
- Fiber: 1.6
- Total Carbohydrate: 13.5
- Protein: 2.4
- Total Fat: 3.2
- Saturated Fat: 0.3

157. Healthy Banana Oat Muffins

Serving: 9-12 muffins, 12 serving(s) | Prep: 10mins | Ready in:

Ingredients

- 3 mashed bananas
- 2 tablespoons unsweetened applesauce
- 1 egg
- 1/2 cup nonfat milk
- 3/4 teaspoon vanilla extract
- 2/3 cup whole wheat flour
- 1/2 cup quick-cooking oats
- 2 tablespoons Splenda sugar substitute
- 1 3/4 teaspoons baking powder
- 3/4 teaspoon ground cinnamon
- 1/4 teaspoon salt
- 2 tablespoons ground flax seeds (optional)
- walnuts (optional)

Direction

- Preheat oven to 375.
- Combine bananas and next 4 ingredients (through vanilla) in a medium bowl; mix well and set aside.
- Lightly spoon flour into a dry measuring cup and level with a knife. Whisk together flour and next 6 ingredients (through flaxseed if used) in small bowl.
- Stir the flour mixture into the banana mixture until they are just combined.
- Spray 12 muffin cups (for smaller muffins) or 9 muffin cups (for larger muffins) with cooking spray (or use paper liners) and spoon just about 1/4°C batter into each cup for 12 muffins.
- Sprinkle muffin batter with some chopped walnuts.
- Bake 18 minutes.

Nutrition Information

- Calories: 74.1
- Saturated Fat: 0.2
- Protein: 2.7
- Total Carbohydrate: 15
- Cholesterol: 17.8
- Total Fat: 0.9
- Sodium: 113.4
- Fiber: 2
- Sugar: 4.3

158. Healthy Banana And Chocolate Chip Muffins

Serving: 14-16 serving(s) | Prep: 15mins | Ready in:

Ingredients

- 4 bananas, very ripe
- 1/2 cup brown sugar
- 3 tablespoons maple syrup
- 2 eggs
- 2 teaspoons baking soda
- 2 teaspoons baking powder
- 1/2 teaspoon salt
- 1 1/2 cups flour
- 1 cup oats
- 4 ounces applesauce
- 1 teaspoon vanilla
- 1 teaspoon cinnamon
- 1 cup chocolate chips

Direction

- Preheat the oven to 400 degrees.
- Spray two muffin tins with canola oil.
- In a large mixing bowl, mash the bananas with a fork.
- Add the sugar and maple syrup and mix well with the fork.
- Add the eggs and beat those into the banana mixture still using the fork.
- Add the dry ingredients and mix well.
- Then add the applesauce, vanilla and cinnamon and chocolate chips and mix again.
- Pour into the muffin tins and bake for 12-14 minutes.

Nutrition Information

- Calories: 238.7
- Total Fat: 5.3
- Saturated Fat: 2.5
- Sodium: 332.7
- Fiber: 3.3
- Cholesterol: 30.2
- Sugar: 20.9
- Total Carbohydrate: 45.4
- Protein: 5.1

159. Healthy Berry Muffins

Serving: 9 muffins | Prep: 20mins | Ready in:

Ingredients

- 1 cup oats
- 3/4 cup low-fat sour cream
- 100 g low-fat berry yogurt (or one small container)
- 2/3 cup brown sugar
- 1 egg
- 1 cup flour
- 1/4 teaspoon salt
- 1/2 teaspoon baking soda
- 1 teaspoon baking powder
- 3/4 cup frozen mixed berries (or fresh)

Direction

- Mix oats, sour cream and yogurt and let stand for 15 minutes.
- Sift and mix together flour, salt, baking soda and baking powder.
- Add in egg and brown sugar to oats mixture.
- Incorporate dry ingredients to oats mixture.
- Mix in berries.
- Fill greased muffin tins.
- Bake at 400° for 20 minutes for large muffins or 15 minutes for mini muffins.
- (Makes about 9 large muffins or 12 mini muffins).

Nutrition Information

- Calories: 226.7
- Sodium: 202.7
- Fiber: 2.2
- Protein: 6.2
- Cholesterol: 29
- Total Fat: 4.4
- Saturated Fat: 2
- Sugar: 18
- Total Carbohydrate: 41.2

160. Healthy Blueberry Muffins A Nigella Lawson Makeover

Serving: 12 muffins, 6 serving(s) | Prep: 10mins | Ready in:

Ingredients

- 4 tablespoons canola oil
- 1 1/3 cups whole wheat flour
- 1/4 cup Splenda brown sugar blend
- 1/2 teaspoon baking soda
- 2 teaspoons baking powder
- 1 pinch salt
- 1 cup nonfat yogurt
- 1 egg
- 1 cup frozen blueberries
- 1 orange, zest of

Direction

- Preheat oven to 400°F.
- Combine the dry ingredients in a large bowl.
- Whisk wet ingredients in a separate smaller bowl.
- Pour wet into dry and combine - but do not over work.
- Add the orange zest.

- Fold in blueberries.
- Spoon into greased 12-muffin pan.
- Bake for 20 minutes.
- Enjoy!

Nutrition Information

- Calories: 270.8
- Cholesterol: 31.8
- Sugar: 14.5
- Sodium: 296.8
- Fiber: 3.7
- Total Carbohydrate: 38.9
- Protein: 7.1
- Total Fat: 10.9
- Saturated Fat: 1.1

161. Healthy Blueberry Scones

Serving: 24 serving(s) | Prep: 10mins | Ready in:

Ingredients

- 1 cup all-purpose flour
- 1 cup whole wheat flour
- 1/3 cup sugar
- 2 teaspoons baking powder
- 1/2 teaspoon baking soda
- 1/4 teaspoon salt
- 4 tablespoons butter substitute
- 1 egg
- 3/4 cup low-fat buttermilk
- 1 teaspoon vanilla
- 1 cup blueberries

Direction

- Preheat oven to 375 degrees.
- Line a large baking sheet with a silicone mat or parchment paper.
- Combine flour, sugar, baking powder, baking soda and salt in a large bowl. Cut butter into flour mixture with a pastry blender or two knives until it resembles a coarse crumbs.
- Add egg, buttermilk and vanilla. Stir with a fork until a dough forms. Fold in blueberries. Drop by tablespoonfuls onto prepared baking sheet.
- Bake for 12-14 minutes.
- Yield 24 small scones.

Nutrition Information

- Calories: 57
- Protein: 1.8
- Total Fat: 0.5
- Sodium: 92
- Fiber: 0.8
- Sugar: 3.8
- Total Carbohydrate: 11.7
- Cholesterol: 8.1
- Saturated Fat: 0.1

162. Healthy Bran Muffins

Serving: 24 Muffins | Prep: 5mins | Ready in:

Ingredients

- 2 1/4 cups wheat bran
- 2 cups milk
- 2 eggs
- 1/4 cup vegetable oil
- 1/2 cup honey, to taste
- 2 1/2 cups flour
- 2 1/2 tablespoons baking powder
- 1 teaspoon salt
- 1 teaspoon cinnamon
- 1 1/2 cups raisins
- 3/4 cup walnuts or 3/4 cup pecans, chopped (optional)

Direction

- In a large mixing bowl combine the bran, milk, eggs, oil and honey.
- In a second bowl, combine all the remaining ingredients.

- Add the dry mixture to the liquid and mix thoroughly.
- Fill oiled muffin tins.
- Bake in 350 F degree oven for 30 minutes, or until tops are lightly browned.
- Cool on a rack.
- When thoroughly cooled, store covered in refrigerator or freezer.

Nutrition Information

- Calories: 171.8
- Fiber: 3.3
- Sugar: 11.3
- Total Carbohydrate: 28.3
- Total Fat: 6.2
- Saturated Fat: 1.2
- Sodium: 227.9
- Cholesterol: 20.5
- Protein: 4.2

163. Healthy Chocolate/Berry Muffins

Serving: 12 muffins, 12 serving(s) | Prep: 10mins | Ready in:

Ingredients

- 1 cup yogurt, plain or 1 cup vanilla
- 1 cup rolled oats
- 1/2 cup all-purpose flour
- 1/2 cup whole wheat flour
- 1 teaspoon baking powder
- 1/2 teaspoon baking soda
- 2/3 cup brown sugar
- 1 egg
- 1 teaspoon vanilla
- 1/2 cup oil
- 1 cup chocolate chips or 1 cup berries

Direction

- Preheat oven to 350 degrees.
- Mix yogurt and oats and set aside to moisten.
- Combine flours, baking powder, baking soda and brown sugar.
- Add egg, vanilla, oil, and oat/yoghurt mixture. Mix well to combine.
- Add 1 cup of chocolate chips or berries. Mix again.
- Divide into 12 paper lined muffin tin.
- Bake 20 to 25 minutes.

Nutrition Information

- Calories: 275.1
- Total Fat: 14.9
- Sodium: 104.9
- Fiber: 2.2
- Saturated Fat: 4.3
- Sugar: 20.6
- Total Carbohydrate: 34
- Cholesterol: 20.3
- Protein: 4.1

164. Healthy Cottage Cheese Muffins

Serving: 6 muffins, 4-6 serving(s) | Prep: 5mins | Ready in:

Ingredients

- 1/2 cup flour (any kind will do)
- 1/4 teaspoon salt
- 1 teaspoon baking powder
- 1 egg, beaten
- 1/2 cup cottage cheese, low-fat
- 1 tablespoon vegetable oil
- 1 tablespoon honey
- 1 tablespoon sugar (as much or little as you desire)

Direction

- Preheat oven to 400 deg F/200 deg Celsius.
- Grease muffin pan/line with muffin cups.

- Mix flour, salt and baking powder together.
- In a separate bowl, beat the egg and then beat in cottage cheese. Stir in vegetable oil and honey. Mix well.
- Add wet ingredients into dry ingredients. Mix lightly with a fork. Do not overmix; batter should still be lumpy.
- Pour batter into muffin cups.
- Sprinkle some sugar onto the tops of the unbaked muffins.
- Bake for 15-20 minutes, or until knife to the center comes out clean, or until golden brown.
- Remove from oven immediately and place on wire rack.
- Immediately sprinkle some sugar onto the tops of the muffins and allow to rest for 5-10 minutes.
- Note: The muffins themselves are not very sweet, so the sugar should be added according to how sweet you like your food.

Nutrition Information

- Calories: 159.3
- Saturated Fat: 1.3
- Sodium: 350
- Fiber: 0.4
- Total Carbohydrate: 20.6
- Cholesterol: 51
- Total Fat: 5.9
- Sugar: 8.2
- Protein: 6.1

165. Healthy Ginger Carrot Muffins

Serving: 12 serving(s) | Prep: 15mins | Ready in:

Ingredients

- 1 1/2 cups whole wheat flour
- 2 teaspoons baking soda
- 2 teaspoons cinnamon
- 1 teaspoon ginger
- 1 teaspoon clove
- 1 teaspoon nutmeg
- 2 tablespoons ground flax seeds
- 2 large egg whites
- 1 cup sugar substitute (I use Splenda)
- 1/4 cup molasses
- 1/4 cup unsweetened applesauce
- 1/3 cup soymilk (I use Silk)
- 3 cups shredded carrots, packed or 1 (16 ounce) bag baby carrots, finely chopped in food processor
- 1 1/4 cups old fashioned oats

Direction

- Preheat oven to 350°F.
- Sift together flour, baking soda, cinnamon, ginger, cloves, and nutmeg. Add ground flaxseed. Set aside.
- In large mixing bowl, beat egg whites until foamy. Add Splenda, molasses, soymilk, and applesauce until smooth.
- Stir in carrots.
- Gradually add flour mixture to carrot mixture.
- Stir in oats.
- Fill muffin cups 2/3 full.
- Bake for 15-20 minutes.
- Enjoy!

Nutrition Information

- Calories: 183.9
- Total Fat: 1.6
- Cholesterol: 0
- Protein: 5.1
- Saturated Fat: 0.3
- Sodium: 246.4
- Fiber: 4.2
- Sugar: 16.8
- Total Carbohydrate: 38.8

166. Healthy Mystery Muffins

Serving: 12 cupcakes | Prep: 10mins | Ready in:

Ingredients

- 1 (18 1/4 ounce) package devil's food cake mix
- 15 ounces pumpkin
- pecans, a handful at a time chopped
- chocolate chips, a handful at a
- 1 tablespoon vanilla

Direction

- Preheat oven to 350 degrees.
- Grease 12 muffin cups or line with paper baking cups.
- Mix cake mix with pumpkin.
- Add vanilla.
- Drop into cupcake tins and sprinkle with chopped pecans and chocolate chips.
- Bake for 20 minutes.

Nutrition Information

- Calories: 196.9
- Saturated Fat: 1.4
- Fiber: 1.2
- Total Carbohydrate: 33.9
- Cholesterol: 0
- Total Fat: 6.8
- Sodium: 356.2
- Sugar: 17.1
- Protein: 2.9

167. Healthy Prune Oatmeal Muffins

Serving: 6-12 serving(s) | Prep: 5mins | Ready in:

Ingredients

- 3/4 cup all-purpose flour
- 1/4 cup oat flour
- 1 tablespoon wheat germ
- 1/4 cup Splenda sugar substitute
- 1 1/2 teaspoons baking powder
- 1 teaspoon salt
- 1/2 teaspoon baking soda
- 1 1/3 cups oats (quick rolled)
- 1 cup prune, pitted and chopped
- 1 cup low-fat buttermilk
- 1/4 cup light butter, softened
- 1/4 cup molasses
- 1 large egg

Direction

- Preheat oven to 400 degrees.
- Mix together the flours, Splenda baking powder, salt, wheat germ, and soda. Stir in the oats and prunes.
- Add the buttermilk, butter, molasses, and egg, and stir till mixed. Batter will resemble cake batter. Pour into a nonstick muffin tin. Either 6 large muffin size, or 12 small size. Bake until lightly brown and springy. Turn muffins out of pan and allow to cool. Delicious warm or cold.

Nutrition Information

- Calories: 333.2
- Total Fat: 8.2
- Fiber: 4.9
- Sugar: 21.1
- Cholesterol: 47.1
- Protein: 8.7
- Saturated Fat: 4.1
- Sodium: 688.8
- Total Carbohydrate: 59

168. Healthy Spiced Butternut Squash Muffins

Serving: 12 serving(s) | Prep: 10mins | Ready in:

Ingredients

- 3/4 cup butternut squash, cooked and pureed (original calls for 1 cup)
- 1 1/2 cups white whole wheat flour

- 2 teaspoons baking powder
- 1/3 cup white sugar
- 1/4 teaspoon salt
- 1 teaspoon cinnamon
- 1/4 teaspoon nutmeg
- 1/4 teaspoon clove
- 1/4 teaspoon ginger
- 3/4 cup milk
- 1 egg, beaten
- 1 tablespoon butter, melted
- cinnamon baking chips (optional)
- chocolate chips (optional)

Direction

- Preheat oven to 400 degrees F (200 degrees C). Lightly grease a 12 cup muffin pan.
- In a large bowl, whisk together flour, baking powder, white sugar, salt and pumpkin pie spice.
- In a medium bowl, thoroughly mix together milk, egg and butter. Stir in squash. Fold the squash mixture into the flour mixture just until moistened.
- Spoon the batter into the prepared muffin pan, filling cups about 1/2 full.
- If desired, drop a few chocolate chips or cinnamon chips on top of the batter.
- Bake 20 minutes in the preheated oven, or until a toothpick inserted in the center of a muffin comes out clean. Remove from muffin pan and cool on a wire rack.

Nutrition Information

- Calories: 102.1
- Total Fat: 2.3
- Saturated Fat: 1.2
- Total Carbohydrate: 18.6
- Sodium: 131.7
- Fiber: 1.9
- Sugar: 5.8
- Cholesterol: 20.2
- Protein: 3.1

169. Healthy W.w Oatmeal Raisin Muffins

Serving: 12 muffins, 12-15 serving(s) | Prep: 10mins | Ready in:

Ingredients

- 1 1/4 cups whole wheat flour
- 1 1/2 cups oats
- 1/3 cup date syrup (more to add sweetness)
- 2 teaspoons baking soda
- 2 teaspoons cinnamon (possibly even more)
- 1/4 teaspoon salt
- 3/4 cup water
- 1/4 cup soymilk
- 1/4 cup applesauce
- 1 egg
- 1/2 cup raisins

Direction

- Preheat oven to 350. Line muffin tin with cupcake holders. Mix dry ingredients in a large bowl. Combine wet ingredients in a separate bowl. Add wet ingredients to the dry ingredients. Does not need too much mixing. Add raisins last. Pour into cupcake holders about 3/4 full. Bake for 10 to 15 minutes. Until they are moist but not wet. Take out of tin and cool on a cooling rack. It is much better room temperature.

Nutrition Information

- Calories: 150.1
- Total Carbohydrate: 28.4
- Fiber: 4.2
- Sodium: 270.4
- Sugar: 3.7
- Cholesterol: 17.6
- Protein: 6
- Total Fat: 2.1
- Saturated Fat: 0.4

170. Healthy, Moist Bran Muffins

Serving: 18 muffins, 18 serving(s) | Prep: 10mins | Ready in:

Ingredients

- 2 1/4 cups all-bran cereal
- 1/2 cup raisins
- 1 cup all-purpose flour
- 3/4 cup whole wheat flour
- 1/2 cup packed light brown sugar
- 2 teaspoons baking soda
- 1/2 teaspoon salt
- 6 tablespoons margarine, melted
- 2 large eggs
- 1 3/4 cups plain yogurt
- 1/4 cup unsulphured molasses
- 2 teaspoons vanilla extract
- optional sugar crystals

Direction

- Preheat the oven to 400 degrees F. In a food processor, finely grind half of the cereal. Add the raisins to the mixture, but do not grind them. Transfer the mixture to a bowl with remaining cereal, flour, whole-wheat flour, sugar, baking soda, and salt. Set aside.
- Combine butter, eggs, yogurt, molasses, and vanilla. Stir together wet and dry ingredients until just combined. Do not over mix.
- Line muffin tin with baking cups. Fill each just more than halfway. Sprinkle generously with sugar crystals, if desired (they add a good taste). Bake until muffins spring back when touched or when a toothpick inserted into the center comes out clean, about 18 minutes. Remove from tin and allow to cool slightly.

Nutrition Information

- Calories: 168.9
- Sodium: 291.9
- Fiber: 3.1
- Protein: 4.1
- Total Fat: 5.7
- Saturated Fat: 1.5
- Sugar: 13.4
- Total Carbohydrate: 28.6
- Cholesterol: 23.8

171. Hedgehog Biscuits

Serving: 24 Hedgehogs | Prep: 30mins | Ready in:

Ingredients

- 125 g unsalted butter
- 1 cup icing sugar
- 2 tablespoons cocoa
- 1 egg, lightly beaten
- 1/4 cup coconut
- 2 cups Marie biscuits (for Australians) or 2 cups graham crackers, broken into pieces (for Americans)
- 1/2 cup hazelnuts
- Icing
- 125 g dark chocolate
- 125 g milk chocolate
- 1 tablespoon Copha

Direction

- Melt the butter in a large saucepan over a medium heat.
- Remove the pan from the heat, and stir in the sifted icing sugar and cocoa, and mix well.
- Stir in the beaten egg, and return the pan to the heat and stir until the mixture boils.
- Remove the pan from the heat and stir in the coconut, biscuit pieces and nuts. The biscuits are generally broken into pieces about the size of a hazelnut, but some larger pieces is fine, and the pieces certainly don't have to all be the same size!
- Spoon the mixture into a baking paper lined 18cm x 28cm (approximately 7" x 11") slice pan and press down firmly.

- Icing the Hedgehogs: Melt the dark chocolate, milk chocolate and copha together in a microwave-safe bowl or jug in a microwave oven on a Medium setting for approximately 2 minutes; stir well, pour - and spread evenly - over the hedgehog base.
- Chill to set.
- Once chilled, cut into 24 slices. Or larger or smaller slices if you wish!
- Notes: For extra flavour, add 1/4 cup of sultanas.

Nutrition Information

- Calories: 147.9
- Fiber: 1.7
- Cholesterol: 21.2
- Total Fat: 12
- Sodium: 9.4
- Sugar: 7.8
- Total Carbohydrate: 10.8
- Protein: 2
- Saturated Fat: 6.6

172. High Protein, High Fiber Blueberry Muffins

Serving: 12 Muffins, 12 serving(s) | Prep: 10mins | Ready in:

Ingredients

- 1 cup soy flour
- 1 cup quick oats
- 1 cup wheat bran (I use quaker natural bran flakes)
- 1/2 cup whole wheat flour
- 1/2 cup ground flax seeds
- 2 teaspoons cream of tartar
- 1 teaspoon baking soda
- 2 tablespoons cinnamon
- 4 egg whites
- 1 cup 1% low-fat milk
- 3/4 cup low-fat plain yogurt (I use organic Balkan style)
- 1/4 cup honey (or cane sugar)
- 1 cup frozen blueberries

Direction

- Preheat oven to 400 degrees. Spray a 12 cup muffin tin with non-stick cooking spray.
- Combine all dry ingredients in a large bowl and make a well in the middle.
- Combine all wet ingredients in another bowl and mix well.
- Pour wet ingredients into well and mix slightly. Add berries and mix until just combined. Don't over mix.
- Fill muffin cups equally with batter and bake for 20 minutes. Remove from oven and cool.

Nutrition Information

- Calories: 180.4
- Saturated Fat: 0.8
- Fiber: 5.7
- Sugar: 13.9
- Total Carbohydrate: 30
- Cholesterol: 1.6
- Total Fat: 4.7
- Sodium: 144.9
- Protein: 8.8

173. Holiday Gingerbread Muffins

Serving: 12 muffins | Prep: 10mins | Ready in:

Ingredients

- 1 egg
- 1/4 cup applesauce
- 3 tablespoons vegetable oil
- 1/4 cup molasses
- 1/2 cup sugar
- 1 1/2 cups flour

- 1 teaspoon baking soda
- 1/2 teaspoon salt
- 1 teaspoon cinnamon
- 1/2 teaspoon clove
- 1/4 teaspoon ginger
- 1/4 teaspoon nutmeg
- 1/2 cup boiling water
- sugar, to sprinkle

Direction

- Preheat oven to 350°.
- Grease 12 muffin cup/tins.
- In medium bowl, beat the egg, applesauce, oil, molasses and 1/2 cup sugar.
- Combine dry ingredients in a medium bowl and add to first mixture.
- Stir in the water, mixing well.
- Fill the muffin cups two-thirds full.
- Lightly sprinkle with sugar.
- Bake at 350° for 20 to 25 minutes or until done.

Nutrition Information

- Calories: 150.9
- Sodium: 212.5
- Fiber: 0.6
- Sugar: 12.3
- Total Carbohydrate: 26.9
- Protein: 2.2
- Total Fat: 4
- Saturated Fat: 0.6
- Cholesterol: 17.6

174. Homemade Cornbread

Serving: 12 serving(s) | Prep: 10mins | Ready in:

Ingredients

- 1 cup cornmeal
- 1/2 cup all-purpose flour
- 2 teaspoons baking powder
- 2 teaspoons sugar
- 1 cup skim milk
- 1/4 cup egg substitute
- 3 tablespoons canola oil

Direction

- Preheat oven to 425 degrees.
- Prepare an 8X8 baking dish with cooking spray (I prefer Pam).
- In bowl, combine cornmeal, flour, sugar, and baking powder.
- In separate bowl, combine milk, egg substitute, and oil.
- Add the dry ingredients to the wet and stir until slightly moistened.
- Pour batter into baking dish.
- Bake approximately 15 minutes or until slightly brown.

Nutrition Information

- Calories: 102.6
- Total Carbohydrate: 13.8
- Total Fat: 4.1
- Saturated Fat: 0.4
- Fiber: 0.9
- Cholesterol: 0.5
- Protein: 2.8
- Sodium: 85.5
- Sugar: 0.8

175. Homemade Scones

Serving: 1 dozen, 4-6 serving(s) | Prep: 10mins | Ready in:

Ingredients

- 2 cups self raising flour
- 1 teaspoon baking powder
- 1 pinch salt
- 25 g caster sugar
- 50 g butter
- 125 ml milk

- 125 ml water

Direction

- Preheat oven to 220°C.
- Sift together the flour, baking powder and salt into a bowl.
- Stir in the sugar, add the slightly softened butter and rub into the flour until resembling bread crumbs.
- Add nearly all the milk and water mix, a little at a time, working to a smooth dough. Reserve the remaining milk.
- Roll on a lightly floured work surface until 2cm thick.
- Using a 5 cm pastry cutter, cut the dough, using one sharp tap and not twisting the dough as you cut.
- Brush the tops with the remaining milk mixture.
- Place the scones on a greased baking tray and bake in the oven for 10 to 12 minutes, until golden brown.

Nutrition Information

- Calories: 360.9
- Total Carbohydrate: 55.6
- Total Fat: 11.8
- Saturated Fat: 7.2
- Sodium: 217.9
- Sugar: 6.4
- Fiber: 1.7
- Cholesterol: 31
- Protein: 7.6

176. Homestyle Biscuits

Serving: 15 serving(s) | Prep: 15mins | Ready in:

Ingredients

- 2 cups flour
- 2 teaspoons baking powder
- 1/4 teaspoon baking soda
- 1/4 teaspoon salt
- 2 tablespoons sugar
- 2/3 cup 1% fat buttermilk
- 3 1/3 tablespoons vegetable oil

Direction

- Preheat oven to 450 degrees F.
- In medium bowl, combine flour, baking powder, baking soda, salt, and sugar.
- In small bowl, stir together buttermilk and all of the oil. Pour over flour mixture and stir until well mixed.
- On lightly floured surface, knead dough gently for 10 to 12 strokes. Roll or pat dough to 3/4-inch thickness. Cut with 2-inch biscuit or cookie cutter, dipping cutter in flour between cuts. Transfer biscuits to an ungreased baking sheet.
- Bake for 12 minutes or until golden brown. Serve warm.

Nutrition Information

- Calories: 98.5
- Total Fat: 3.3
- Saturated Fat: 0.5
- Sodium: 119.9
- Sugar: 2.2
- Fiber: 0.5
- Total Carbohydrate: 15.1
- Cholesterol: 0.4
- Protein: 2.1

177. Honey Oat Biscuits

Serving: 30 biscuits, 30 serving(s) | Prep: 5mins | Ready in:

Ingredients

- 125 g butter, softened
- 1/2 cup sugar

- 2 tablespoons honey
- 1 cup flour, plain
- 1 teaspoon baking powder (when using Australian BP I use 2 tsp)
- 1/2 teaspoon cinnamon
- 1 1/2 cups rolled oats

Direction

- Cream butter, sugar and honey until pale.
- Sift flour, baking powder and cinnamon together. Add sifted ingredients and rolled oats to creamed mixture, stirring well.
- Roll tablespoonful of mixture into balls.
- Place on greased oven tray and flatten with a floured fork.
- Bake at 180C for 15 minutes or until golden.
- Transfer to a rack to cool.

Nutrition Information

- Calories: 77.5
- Protein: 1
- Total Fat: 3.7
- Saturated Fat: 2.2
- Cholesterol: 8.9
- Sugar: 4.5
- Total Carbohydrate: 10.5
- Sodium: 42.1
- Fiber: 0.6

178. Honey Peach Bran Muffins

Serving: 12 muffins | Prep: 5mins | Ready in:

Ingredients

- 1/2 cup all-purpose flour
- 3/4 cup whole wheat flour
- 1/4 cup wheat bran
- 1 teaspoon baking powder
- 1 teaspoon baking soda
- 1 teaspoon cinnamon
- 1/4 cup honey
- 1 egg white, lightly beaten
- 1 cup peach yogurt
- 1/4 cup vegetable oil
- 1/2 cup drained chopped canned peaches

Direction

- Preheat oven to 350 degrees F.
- Combine flours, bran, baking powder, baking soda, and cinnamon.
- Separately, combine honey, egg white, yogurt, and oil; stir well.
- Pour liquid into dry ingredients; stir until just moistened.
- Add peaches.
- Pour into greased muffin tins.
- Bake at 350 degrees F for 18-20 minutes or until lightly browned.

Nutrition Information

- Calories: 137.2
- Sodium: 152.9
- Fiber: 1.8
- Sugar: 11.2
- Total Carbohydrate: 21.7
- Cholesterol: 0.8
- Protein: 3
- Saturated Fat: 0.8
- Total Fat: 5

179. Honey Rice Muffins

Serving: 12 muffins | Prep: 10mins | Ready in:

Ingredients

- 1 egg
- 1/4 cup honey
- 2 tablespoons oil
- 1/2 cup milk
- 1 teaspoon vanilla
- 1 cup cooked rice

- 1 cup flour
- 1 tablespoon baking powder
- 1/2 teaspoon baking soda
- 1/2 teaspoon salt

Direction

- Mix together the flour, powder, soda and salt.
- Add to the dry ingredients, the egg, honey, oil, milk, vanilla and rice all at once.
- Stir just until blended.
- Spoon into muffin tin.
- Bake at 400 for 15 minutes.

Nutrition Information

- Calories: 113.8
- Saturated Fat: 0.7
- Sugar: 5.9
- Total Fat: 3.2
- Fiber: 0.3
- Total Carbohydrate: 19
- Cholesterol: 19.1
- Protein: 2.3
- Sodium: 251.4

180. Hot Water Cornbread

Serving: 8 patties, 8 serving(s) | Prep: 5mins | Ready in:

Ingredients

- 2 cups white cornmeal
- 1/4 teaspoon baking powder
- 1 1/4 teaspoons salt
- 1 teaspoon sugar
- 1/4 cup half-and-half
- 1 tablespoon vegetable oil
- 3/4-1 1/4 cup boiling water
- vegetable oil
- softened butter

Direction

- Combine first 4 ingredients in a bowl; stir in half and half and 1 tablespoon oil. Gradually add boiling water, stirring until batter is the consistency of grits.
- Pour oil to a depth of 1/2 inch into a large heavy skillet (cast iron), place over medium high heat. Scoop batter into a 1/4 cup measure; drop into hot oil, and fry in batches 3 minutes on each side or until golden. Drain well on paper towels. Serve immediately with softened butter.

Nutrition Information

- Calories: 137.4
- Total Fat: 3.7
- Sugar: 0.7
- Cholesterol: 2.8
- Saturated Fat: 0.9
- Sodium: 388.9
- Fiber: 2.2
- Total Carbohydrate: 24.3
- Protein: 2.7

181. Ina's Cheddar Dill Scones

Serving: 1 large, 16 serving(s) | Prep: 10mins | Ready in:

Ingredients

- 4 cups all-purpose flour, divided
- 1 tablespoon all-purpose flour, divided
- 2 tablespoons baking powder
- 2 teaspoons salt
- 3/4 lb cold unsalted butter, diced
- 4 extra-large eggs, beaten lightly
- 1 cup cold heavy cream
- 1/2 lb extra-sharp yellow cheddar cheese, small-diced
- 1 cup minced fresh dill
- 1 egg (beaten with water or milk, for egg wash)
- 1 tablespoon water (for egg wash) or 1 tablespoon milk (for egg wash)

Direction

- Preheat the oven to 400 degrees F.
- Combine 4 cups of flour, the baking powder, and salt in the bowl of an electric mixer fitted with a paddle attachment. Add the butter and mix on low speed until the butter is in pea-sized pieces. Mix the eggs and heavy cream and quickly add them to the flour-and-butter mixture. Combine until just blended. Toss together the Cheddar, dill, and 1 tablespoon of flour and add them to the dough. Mix until they are almost incorporated.
- Dump the dough onto a well-floured surface and knead it for 1 minute, until the Cheddar and dill are well distributed. Roll the dough 3/4-inch thick. Cut into 4-inch squares and then in half diagonally to make triangles. Brush the tops with egg wash. Bake on a baking sheet lined with parchment paper for 20 to 25 minutes, until the outside is crusty and the inside is fully baked.

Nutrition Information

- Calories: 403.5
- Total Fat: 29.5
- Saturated Fat: 17.9
- Fiber: 0.9
- Total Carbohydrate: 25.4
- Cholesterol: 155.6
- Sodium: 548.5
- Sugar: 0.3
- Protein: 9.5

182. Italian Biscuits

Serving: 12 9-12 biscuits, 4-5 serving(s) | Prep: 15mins | Ready in:

Ingredients

- 2 cups baking mix, Bisquick recommended
- 2/3 cup whole milk
- 2/3 cup parmesan cheese, grated
- 1 cup pepperoni, chopped
- 1 1/2 teaspoons parsley, chopped and divided
- 1 teaspoon garlic powder, divided
- 1/4 cup butter

Direction

- Mix together the Baking Mix, grated Parmesan cheese 1/2 teaspoons garlic powder and one teaspoons parsley until thoroughly combined. Add the chopped Pepperoni and mix together.
- Add 2/3 cup whole milk and mix together with a wooden spoon until full incorporated. Batter will be somewhat sticky. Add a bit more milk if mixture is too dry.
- Drop by tablespoons onto a cookie sheet 2 inches apart. (No need to grease the cookie sheet).
- Bake at 450 degrees F. for 8-10 minutes or until the tops are browned.
- Melt the 1/2 stick of butter and add the rest of the parsley and garlic powder. Mix together well.
- When biscuits are done brush the tops with the melted butter mixture coating the tops of all the biscuits.
- Serve.

Nutrition Information

- Calories: 751.7
- Total Fat: 52.1
- Saturated Fat: 21.8
- Sodium: 1947.8
- Fiber: 1.4
- Total Carbohydrate: 43.7
- Sugar: 9.7
- Cholesterol: 109.3
- Protein: 25.8

183. Italian Garlic Biscuits

Serving: 2 biscuits, 5 serving(s) | Prep: 10mins | Ready in:

Ingredients

- 1 (8 ounce) canflaky layer biscuits
- 1/2 cup butter
- 1 teaspoon italian seasoning
- 2 tablespoons minced garlic

Direction

- Preheat oven to 350.
- Melt butter in microwave.
- Mix butter, garlic seasoning in 8X8 square baking pan.
- Coat each biscuit with the butter mixture.
- Bake 18-22 minutes uncovered.
- Makes 10 biscuits.

Nutrition Information

- Calories: 327.9
- Total Carbohydrate: 21.4
- Cholesterol: 50.2
- Total Fat: 25.8
- Sodium: 394.4
- Protein: 3.6
- Saturated Fat: 13.6
- Fiber: 0.8
- Sugar: 1

184. Jalapeno Cheddar Cornbread

Serving: 4 serving(s) | Prep: 3mins | Ready in:

Ingredients

- 1 (8 1/2 ounce) box Jiffy cornbread mix
- 1 egg
- 1/4 cup butter, melted
- 1/3 cup milk
- 2 tablespoons canned jalapeno peppers, diced and drained well
- 1 cup cheddar cheese, shredded
- 1/8 teaspoon salt (optional)

Direction

- Combine cornbread mix, egg and butter in a mixing bowl.
- Add remaining ingredients. Combine well. Mixture will be thick and lumpy.
- Place cornbread in a greased muffin tin, mini muffin tin or 2-quart casserole dish.
- Bake at 375 degrees for 15-20 minutes or until cornbread is golden brown.

Nutrition Information

- Calories: 510.2
- Sugar: 1.1
- Total Carbohydrate: 45.4
- Cholesterol: 110.7
- Protein: 14
- Total Fat: 30.6
- Fiber: 5
- Sodium: 1685.1
- Saturated Fat: 16

185. Jane's Banana Chocolate Chip Muffins

Serving: 12 muffins, 12 serving(s) | Prep: 10mins | Ready in:

Ingredients

- 1 1/2 cups all-purpose flour
- 1 teaspoon baking soda
- 1 teaspoon baking powder
- 1/2 teaspoon salt
- 4 bananas, ripe
- 1 egg, lightly beaten
- 3/4 cup sugar

- 1/3 cup butter, melted
- 1/2 cup chocolate chips

Direction

- In a bowl, mash bananas; add egg, sugar, melted butter and chocolate chips. Stir until moistened.
- In another bowl, sift together dry ingredients; add to banana mixture. Stir with a fork until moistened. Spoon into greased muffin pan. Bake at 375 degrees for 20 minutes.

Nutrition Information

- Calories: 225.2
- Sodium: 284.5
- Total Fat: 7.9
- Saturated Fat: 4.7
- Fiber: 1.9
- Sugar: 21.2
- Total Carbohydrate: 38
- Cholesterol: 29
- Protein: 2.9

186. Jay's Zero Cholesterol Light Muffins

Serving: 12 muffins, 12 serving(s) | Prep: 10mins | Ready in:

Ingredients

- 1 cup oat bran
- 1 cup all-purpose flour
- 1 tablespoon baking powder
- 1/2 teaspoon cinnamon
- 1 cup skim milk
- 1/2 cup banana, mashed and ripe
- 1/2 cup raisins or 1/2 cup apricots (chopped) or 1/2 cup dates or 1/2 cup prunes or 1/2 cup nuts (chopped)
- 1/4 cup canola oil (100% cholesterol free)
- 1/4 cup brown sugar
- 1 egg white

Direction

- Pre-Heat oven to 400 degrees.
- Line 12 muffin cups with paper baking cups. Combine bran, flour, baking powder, cinnamon and sugar in one bowl.
- Combine remaining wet ingredients i.e. milk, banana, chopped fruit, oil, egg white in another bowl.
- Mix dry and wet together, and turn over ingredients lightly just until dry ingredients are moistened.
- Do not stir or beat vigorously.
- Fill prepared muffin cups 3/4 full.
- Bake 20 to 25 minutes or until golden brown.

Nutrition Information

- Calories: 148.9
- Total Fat: 5.3
- Saturated Fat: 0.5
- Cholesterol: 0.4
- Protein: 3.8
- Sodium: 110.5
- Fiber: 1.9
- Sugar: 8.9
- Total Carbohydrate: 25.3

187. Jelly Crystal Biscuits (Cookies)

Serving: 48 cookies | Prep: 10mins | Ready in:

Ingredients

- 100 g butter
- 200 g jelly crystals (I used 2x 85 gram packets)
- 1/4 cup sugar
- 1 egg
- 1 1/2 cups flour
- 1 teaspoon baking powder

Direction

- Preheat oven to 180°C.
- Cream the butter, jelly crystals and sugar together in a mixer.
- Add egg and beat well.
- Add the sifted flour and baking powder and mix until well combined.
- Place in teaspoonful sizes on an oven tray. Flatten slightly with a fork.
- Bake for approximately 10-12 minutes.

Nutrition Information

- Calories: 50.5
- Fiber: 0.1
- Total Carbohydrate: 7.8
- Protein: 0.9
- Total Fat: 1.8
- Saturated Fat: 1.1
- Sodium: 43.3
- Sugar: 4.6
- Cholesterol: 8.3

188. Jen's Easy Apricot, Cream Ginger Scones

Serving: 9 scones | Prep: 10mins | Ready in:

Ingredients

- 2 cups self raising flour
- 1 pinch salt
- 2 teaspoons sugar
- 1/2-1 teaspoon ground ginger (use more if you like)
- 1/2 cup dried apricot (roughly chopped)
- 1/2 cup heavy cream, plus
- 2 tablespoons heavy cream
- 1/2 cup ginger ale, plus
- 2 tablespoons ginger ale

Direction

- Pre heat oven to 400'F/200'C.
- In a bowl mix together all the dry ingredients and stir through the apricot pieces.
- Add in the cream and ginger ale and mix lightly with a knife until mixture holds together in a ball.
- Tip out onto a floured board and gently pat out into a rectangle and cut into 9 scones or cut out scones with a 6cm diameter cutter.
- Place close together on a baking tray lined with baking paper and bake in hot oven for 15 minutes.
- Tip out onto a clean tea towel and wrap up to keep warm.
- These are nice just buttered but even better spread with some apricot jam and topped with a dollop of whipped cream for a special treat.

Nutrition Information

- Calories: 185.3
- Total Fat: 6.4
- Sodium: 26
- Total Carbohydrate: 28.7
- Cholesterol: 22.7
- Protein: 3.5
- Saturated Fat: 3.9
- Fiber: 1.3
- Sugar: 6.4

189. Jim N Nicks Cheese Biscuits

Serving: 12 muffins | Prep: 10mins | Ready in:

Ingredients

- 1 1/2 cups flour
- 1 cup sugar
- 1 cup shredded cheddar cheese
- 3/4 cup milk (2% works best)
- 1 egg, beaten well
- 4 tablespoons butter, softened
- 1 1/2 teaspoons baking powder

- 1/4 teaspoon vanilla

Direction

- Mix all ingredients together. Pour into greased muffin pan and bake at 400 for 15 - 20 minutes.
- This recipe make about 12 muffins.

Nutrition Information

- Calories: 209.5
- Saturated Fat: 4.9
- Sodium: 151.5
- Fiber: 0.4
- Sugar: 16.8
- Total Carbohydrate: 29.6
- Cholesterol: 37.7
- Total Fat: 8.1
- Protein: 5

190. Joyce's Jiffy Corn Muffins

Serving: 12 serving(s) | Prep: 5mins | Ready in:

Ingredients

- 1 (8 1/2 ounce) package Jiffy corn muffin mix
- 1 (9 ounce) packageof jiffy yellow cake mix
- 2 eggs
- 1/3 cup milk
- 1/2 cup water

Direction

- Mix each pkg according to the directions on the packages.
- Combine
- Fill muffin cups 1/2 full
- Bake @375 for 15 minutes or until golden brown.

Nutrition Information

- Calories: 192.4
- Saturated Fat: 1.4
- Sodium: 378
- Fiber: 1.5
- Total Carbohydrate: 30.9
- Total Fat: 6
- Sugar: 13.4
- Cholesterol: 37
- Protein: 3.6

191. KFC Biscuits (Copycat)

Serving: 9-12 serving(s) | Prep: 10mins | Ready in:

Ingredients

- BISCUITS
- 2 cups all-purpose flour
- 1 1/2 teaspoons salt
- 1 tablespoon sugar
- 4 teaspoons baking powder
- 1/4 teaspoon baking soda
- 3 tablespoons vegetable shortening
- 4 teaspoons Butter Flavor Crisco
- 1 cup buttermilk
- BEFORE-BAKING BASTE
- whole milk
- AFTER-BAKING BASTE
- margarine (butter okay)

Direction

- PREHEAT oven to 400°F; COMBINE 2 cups all-purpose flour, 1 1/2 teaspoons salt, 1 tablespoon sugar, 4 teaspoons baking powder and 1/4 teaspoon baking soda in a large mixing bowl; CUT in shortenings until mixture resembles coarse crumbs.
- STIR in 1 cup buttermilk just until a soft dough forms (dough will be very loose and sticky at this point).
- SPRINKLE flour over a large wooden board; TURN dough onto a floured board and knead gently 10 to 12 times or until no longer sticky, re-flouring board as necessary while kneading.

- DIVIDE dough in half; GENTLY pat or roll each half into an 8-inch circle 1/2-inch thick.
- CUT out biscuits – pressing straight down – with a 2-inch biscuit cutter.
- REFORM scraps, working it as little as possible and continue cutting.
- PLACE cut biscuits on an ungreased baking sheet with edges barely touching; BRUSH tops of the biscuits with whole milk.
- BAKE for 15 minutes, or until golden brown.
- IMMEDIATELY brush biscuits with margarine (or butter) after baking.
- SERVE hot and enjoy.

Nutrition Information

- Calories: 173.2
- Saturated Fat: 2.2
- Total Carbohydrate: 24.4
- Protein: 3.8
- Total Fat: 6.7
- Sodium: 613.1
- Fiber: 0.8
- Sugar: 2.8
- Cholesterol: 2.1

192. Kim's Fat Free Mini Pumpkin Muffins

Serving: 48 mini muffins, 48 serving(s) | Prep: 10mins | Ready in:

Ingredients

- 1 cup milk
- 1/2 cup applesauce
- 1 (15 ounce) can pumpkin
- 4 egg whites
- 3 cups all-purpose flour
- 4 teaspoons baking powder
- 1 1/2 teaspoons salt
- 1 1/4 cups granulated sugar
- 1/4 cup brown sugar
- 1 1/4 teaspoons cinnamon
- 1 teaspoon nutmeg
- 1/2 teaspoon allspice
- 1/4 teaspoon ginger

Direction

- Preheat oven to 375 degrees.
- Mix all of the ingredients into a large mixing bowl.
- Stir only until all of the ingredients are moistened.
- Scoop into nonstick or paper-lined mini-muffin tray.
- Bake at 375 for 15 minutes and cool on a wire rack.
- Optional: Add 1 cup of walnuts to the batter or it with icing or confectioners' sugar if desired.

Nutrition Information

- Calories: 62.7
- Fiber: 0.3
- Sugar: 6.5
- Protein: 1.4
- Total Fat: 0.3
- Saturated Fat: 0.1
- Sodium: 111.4
- Total Carbohydrate: 13.8
- Cholesterol: 0.7

193. Kiwi Biscuits

Serving: 15 serving(s) | Prep: 5mins | Ready in:

Ingredients

- 1/2 cup softened butter
- 1/4 cup white sugar
- 2 tablespoons sweetened condensed milk
- 1 tablespoon baking powder
- 1 cup flour
- 3/4 cup chocolate chips

Direction

- Combine butter and sugar until creamy.
- Add milk, and stir.
- Add baking powder and flour and combine until just mixed.
- Add chocolate chips and mix all together.
- Roll dough into balls (golf ball size or smaller) and place on an ungreased cookie sheet.
- Press down with fork tines.
- Bake in a moderate over at 350 and remove when the bottoms become golden brown.

Nutrition Information

- Calories: 146.2
- Total Fat: 9
- Saturated Fat: 5.5
- Total Carbohydrate: 16.6
- Protein: 1.5
- Sodium: 120.5
- Fiber: 0.7
- Sugar: 9.3
- Cholesterol: 17.1

194. Last Minute Gingerbread Muffins

Serving: 3 dozen, 18 serving(s) | Prep: 10mins | Ready in:

Ingredients

- 1 cup shortening
- 1 cup sugar
- 1 cup dark molasses
- 4 eggs
- 2 teaspoons baking soda
- 1 cup buttermilk
- 4 cups all-purpose flour
- 1 tablespoon ground ginger
- 1 teaspoon ground ginger
- 1 teaspoon ground allspice
- 1/2 teaspoon ground nutmeg

Direction

- Cream shortening; gradually add sugar, beating until light and fluffy. Stir in molasses. Add eggs, one at a time, beating well after each addition.
- Dissolve soda in buttermilk.
- Combine flour and spices; add to creamed mixture alternately with buttermilk, beating well after each addition.
- Cover and store in refrigerator until ready to bake. Batter can be kept in the refrigerator for 3 weeks.
- To bake, spoon batter into greased muffin pans, filling 2/3rd's full.
- Bake at 350 degrees for 20 minutes.

Nutrition Information

- Calories: 322.3
- Total Carbohydrate: 47.4
- Cholesterol: 41.9
- Sodium: 177.7
- Fiber: 0.8
- Sugar: 22.3
- Total Fat: 12.9
- Saturated Fat: 3.3
- Protein: 4.8

195. Lemon Apple Oat Muffins

Serving: 12 muffins | Prep: 5mins | Ready in:

Ingredients

- 1 egg
- 1/2 cup milk
- 1/4 cup vegetable oil
- 2 tablespoons bottled lemon juice
- 3/4 cup quick-cooking oats
- 1 1/4 cups unsifted flour
- 1/2 cup firmly packed light brown sugar
- 1 1/2 teaspoons baking powder

- 1 teaspoon baking soda
- 1 teaspoon ground cinnamon
- 1/2 teaspoon salt
- 1/4 teaspoon ground nutmeg
- 1 cup finely chopped golden delicious apple (about 1 medium)
- 1/2 cup chopped nuts
- Lemon Icing
- 1/2 cup powdered sugar
- 1 tablespoon lemon juice
- 1 tablespoon melted margarine or 1 tablespoon butter

Direction

- Preheat oven to 400 degrees.
- Combine oats and dry ingredients together in large bowl.
- In medium bowl, beat egg; stir in milk, oil then lemon juice.
- Add to oat mixture with apples and nuts. Mix only until moistened (batter will be thick).
- Spoon into greased or paper baking cup-lined muffin cups.
- Bake 20 minutes or until golden.
- Combine icing ingredients together to make glaze.
- Spoon Lemon Icing over muffins.
- Remove from pan.
- Cool completely.

Nutrition Information

- Calories: 223.3
- Cholesterol: 19.1
- Protein: 4.1
- Sodium: 312
- Fiber: 1.7
- Total Carbohydrate: 31.2
- Sugar: 15.3
- Total Fat: 9.7
- Saturated Fat: 1.6

196. Lemon Cranberry Oat Scones

Serving: 4-6 Scones, 4-6 serving(s) | Prep: 10mins | Ready in:

Ingredients

- 2/3 cup flour
- 2/3 cup oats
- 2 teaspoons baking powder
- 1 tablespoon lemon zest, freshly grated (more, to taste)
- 1 tablespoon sugar (use more if you like your scones sweet)
- 1 tablespoon oil
- 1 cup fresh cranberries or 1 cup frozen cranberries
- 1/4 cup sliced almonds
- 1 teaspoon vanilla extract or 1 teaspoon vanilla powder
- 1/2-2/3 cup milk
- coarse sugar, for sprinkling on top (optional)

Direction

- Heat oven to 400 degrees Fahrenheit.
- Mix dry ingredients together (flour, oats, baking powder, lemon zest, sugar).
- Stir oil into dry ingredients.
- Mix in cranberries and almonds.
- Add vanilla extract and milk.
- Stir until the dry ingredients are damp and will clump together.
- Drop into four mounds (six if you like your scones smaller) on parchment paper lined or greased baking sheet.
- Sprinkle with course sugar, if using.
- Bake for 20 minutes, until lightly browned.

Nutrition Information

- Calories: 287.9
- Protein: 8.9
- Total Fat: 9.5
- Sodium: 198.1
- Fiber: 5.2

- Sugar: 4.6
- Total Carbohydrate: 42.7
- Cholesterol: 4.3
- Saturated Fat: 1.7

197. Lemon Muffins With Toasted Coconut Refreshingly Sweet!

Serving: 15 serving(s) | Prep: 0S | Ready in:

Ingredients

- 15 ounces French vanilla cake mix
- 1 lemon
- 1 tablespoon lemon juice
- 1 teaspoon vanilla extract
- 1 -2 cup powdered sugar (for the glaze)
- 2 tablespoons lemon juice (for the glaze) or 1 tablespoon you can use lemon for a more natural flavor, juice Anjou pear (for the glaze)

Direction

- Follow the directions of the cake mix and have that ready.
- Add 1 tablespoon of lemon juice; grate 1 lemon's zest in there as well. Squeeze 1/2 a lemon's juice also. If you like more lemon flavor you can juice the other half as well.
- Add 1 teaspoon vanilla extract; stir everything together with the cake mix.
- Pour batter into your cake mold of choice- I usually use a loaf pan!
- Bake according to directions on the cake mix box. (Takes about 10-15 minutes).
- Check center using a tooth pick or a fork after 15-20 min to make sure it is baked all the way through. The toothpick should be clean when you enter it into the cake rather than have raw batter on it.
- Once baked through; take muffins out and let them cool.
- Work on making the glaze! Just add the 2 cups of powdered sugar with 2 tablespoons of lemon juice either fresh or from concentrate and mix very well till you get a nice semi-thick consistency. Place aside.
- Once muffins are cool; poke a few tiny openings on top and pour the glaze over them with a spoon. This way the cake absorbs more moisture and the top has a lightly gloss look! Make sure to have aluminum foil or wax paper at the bottom of the cupcakes before pouring the glaze all over. Easier clean up.
- Garnish by grating some lemon zest over the glaze. Your muffins are ready to enjoy!
- Toasted Coconut Portion.
- *Now, if you would like to have an extra depth of flavor to these muffins you can add toasted coconut into the cake batter and garnish with toasted coconut as well. You can buy toasted coconut already packaged or you can toast them yourself. Buy coconut flakes and spread them onto a silicone mat in your pan and place in a 325 degree oven for 3-4 minutes on each side till golden brown!
- Of course, you can make this recipe into a cake or a loaf; it doesn't have to be cupcakes or muffins!

Nutrition Information

- Calories: 156.4
- Sodium: 186.9
- Fiber: 0.4
- Sugar: 20.3
- Cholesterol: 0.6
- Protein: 1.3
- Saturated Fat: 0.5
- Total Carbohydrate: 30.8
- Total Fat: 3.3

198. Lemon And Mango Muffins

Serving: 12 muffins | Prep: 10mins | Ready in:

Ingredients

- 3 cups self rising flour
- 1/2 cup sugar
- 1 teaspoon ground ginger (optional)
- 1 egg, lightly beaten
- 1 lemon, juice and zest of, grated
- 1 1/2 cups buttermilk
- 100 g butter, melted and cooled
- 425 g sliced mangoes in syrup, drained and chopped
- 1/4 cup caster sugar

Direction

- Preheat oven to 220°C.
- Sift the flour, sugar and ginger into a bowl, make a well in the centre.
- Combine the egg, lemon juice, rind and buttermilk. Stir into the dry ingredients, alternatively with melted butter and Mango Slices.
- Divide evenly between 12 greased muffin tins, sprinkle with castor sugar.
- Bake for 15-18 minutes or until well risen and cooked.
- Leave in the tins for 5 minutes before turning onto a wire rack to cool.

Nutrition Information

- Calories: 237.8
- Total Fat: 7.7
- Saturated Fat: 4.6
- Protein: 4.7
- Sugar: 14.2
- Total Carbohydrate: 37.5
- Cholesterol: 36.7
- Sodium: 482.6
- Fiber: 0.9

199. Lemonade Scones

Serving: 8 scones, 8 serving(s) | Prep: 10mins | Ready in:

Ingredients

- 2 cups self raising flour
- 1/4 cup caster sugar
- 1/2 teaspoon salt
- 125 ml lemonade (7 up or Sprite)
- 125 ml whipping cream

Direction

- Preheat oven to 220C degrees.
- Place dry ingredients into a large mixing bowl and combine well.
- Add cream and lemonade and mix to form a soft dough.
- Turn out onto a floured board and knead lightly.
- Press dough gently with your hands and pat until it is approximately 3/4 inch thick.
- Using a round cutter cut out 8 scones.
- Arrange on baking tray, brushing tops with a little milk.
- Bake for 10-15 minutes until tops are lightly browned.

Nutrition Information

- Calories: 197.5
- Protein: 3.5
- Total Fat: 5.8
- Sugar: 8.4
- Fiber: 0.9
- Total Carbohydrate: 32.6
- Cholesterol: 20.4
- Saturated Fat: 3.5
- Sodium: 152.1

200. Light Moist Rhubarb Muffins

Serving: 12-18 muffins | Prep: 10mins | Ready in:

Ingredients

- Muffins
- 2 1/4 cups flour (I use whole wheat flour)
- 1 cup brown sugar
- 1 teaspoon baking soda
- 1 teaspoon baking powder
- 1/2 cup oil
- 1 egg
- 1 teaspoon vanilla
- 1 cup buttermilk (or regular milk with 1 tsp of vinegar or lemon juice that has sat for about 3 minutes)
- 1/2 chopped pecans (optional)
- 1 1/2 cups rhubarb
- Topping
- 1 teaspoon melted butter
- 1/3 cup brown sugar
- 1 teaspoon cinnamon

Direction

- Preheat oven to 400.
- Mix topping ingredients.
- Mix muffin ingredients and fill muffin tin (You can make 12 larger muffins or 18 smaller ones. To avoid a mess of overflowed muffins, try the larger quantity to see how the recipe works out for you and adjust accordingly.)
- Sprinkle topping over muffins.
- Bake for 15 minutes or until a toothpick comes out clean.

Nutrition Information

- Calories: 279.7
- Saturated Fat: 1.7
- Sodium: 175.3
- Fiber: 1
- Protein: 3.8
- Cholesterol: 19.3
- Total Fat: 10.3
- Sugar: 24.8
- Total Carbohydrate: 43.7

201. Light And Fluffy Vegan Lemon Scones

Serving: 8-12 scones, 8-12 serving(s) | Prep: 10mins | Ready in:

Ingredients

- 3 cups all-purpose flour (or whole wheat pastry flour for soft scones)
- 2 tablespoons baking powder
- 1/2 cup sugar
- 1/2 teaspoon salt
- 1/3 cup sunflower oil
- 1 1/2 cups unsweetened soymilk
- 2 teaspoons lemon extract

Direction

- Sift all the dry ingredients together in a bowl, and the wet ingredients in another.
- Combine the wet ingredients into the dry ingredients, mix well but do not over mix-- it's okay if it's a little dry, but add some more soymilk if mix is still left.
- Roll out pieces of the dough onto a cookie sheet covered in parchment paper, you'll get about 8-12 scones.
- Bake at 400F for about 15 minutes or until the tops are firm.

Nutrition Information

- Calories: 327.4
- Total Fat: 10.4
- Sodium: 443.9
- Fiber: 1.9
- Sugar: 12.8
- Cholesterol: 0
- Protein: 6.9

- Saturated Fat: 1.4
- Total Carbohydrate: 51.4

202. Lighter, But Scrumptious Oatmeal Raisin Muffins :)

Serving: 12 serving(s) | Prep: 15mins | Ready in:

Ingredients

- 1 cup oats
- 1 cup skim milk
- 1/2 cup all-purpose flour
- 1/2 cup wheat flour
- 1 teaspoon baking powder
- 1 teaspoon baking soda
- 1 dash salt
- 1 teaspoon cinnamon (optional)
- 1 eggs or 2 egg whites
- 1/2 cup sugar
- 1/2 cup applesauce
- 1 teaspoon vanilla extract
- 1/2-2/3 cup raisins

Direction

- Preheat oven to 375 degrees Fahrenheit.
- Spray 12 cup muffin pan.
- Combine oats and milk in a small bowl, let stand.
- Sift together the flours and all dry ingredients.
- Mix together the egg, sugar, applesauce, and vanilla.
- Mix the oats and milk mixture into the egg mixture.
- Fold in the dry ingredients.
- Fold in raisins.
- Transfer into prepared pan.
- Bake 15 to 20 minutes for muffin tin.
- Take out, ENJOY!

Nutrition Information

- Calories: 160.5
- Total Fat: 1.6
- Sodium: 170.3
- Total Carbohydrate: 32.7
- Cholesterol: 15.9
- Protein: 4.9
- Saturated Fat: 0.4
- Fiber: 2.4
- Sugar: 12

203. Low Fat Banana Chocolate Chip Muffins

Serving: 12-16 serving(s) | Prep: 10mins | Ready in:

Ingredients

- 1 cup sugar
- 1 egg
- 2 ripe bananas, mashed
- 1/3 cup unsweetened applesauce
- 8 ounces low-fat vanilla yogurt or 8 ounces nonfat vanilla yogurt
- 10 ounces semi-sweet chocolate chips
- 2 cups all-purpose flour
- 1 teaspoon baking powder
- 1 teaspoon baking soda
- 1/2 teaspoon salt

Direction

- Combine sugar and egg and blend well.
- Add the mashed bananas, applesauce, and yogurt and stir to combine.
- Stir in chocolate chips and set aside.
- In another bowl, combine the flour, baking powder, baking soda, and salt.
- Add to the wet mixture and stir until just blended- the batter will be lumpy.
- Pour the batter into muffins tins.
- Bake at 375 for 10-15 minutes- be careful not to let them get too brown.

Nutrition Information

- Calories: 287.3
- Total Fat: 7.9
- Fiber: 2.5
- Cholesterol: 18
- Protein: 4.3
- Saturated Fat: 4.4
- Sodium: 246.7
- Sugar: 33.2
- Total Carbohydrate: 54

204. Low Fat Banana Muffins

Serving: 24 serving(s) | Prep: 10mins | Ready in:

Ingredients

- 1 1/4 cups mashed ripe bananas
- 3/4 cup sugar
- 2/3 cup buttermilk
- 4 1/2 tablespoons margarine
- 1/2 teaspoon vanilla extract
- 2 eggs
- 2 2/3 cups all-purpose flour
- 3/4 teaspoon baking powder
- 1 teaspoon baking soda
- 1 teaspoon cinnamon
- 1/4 teaspoon salt
- 1 tablespoon cinnamon
- 4 tablespoons sugar

Direction

- Preheat oven to 350° F.
- Lightly grease muffin tins or line with paper cups.
- Place bananas, sugar, yogurt, melted butter, vanilla, and eggs together in a large mixing bowl and beat with a wooden spoon until smooth.
- In a second bowl sift together flour, baking powder, baking soda, cinnamon and salt.
- Add dry ingredients to wet and mix until just combines. Do not over-mix, or the muffins will be tough.
- Fill muffin cups three-quarters of the way full.
- Mix cinnamon and sugar and sprinkle on to the tops of the muffins to your liking.
- Bake in oven for about 25 minutes.
- A toothpick inserted in the centre of the muffins will come out clean when they are cooked.
- Remove from the oven and cool before serving.

Nutrition Information

- Calories: 118.9
- Fiber: 0.8
- Total Carbohydrate: 21.5
- Total Fat: 2.8
- Saturated Fat: 0.6
- Sodium: 126.5
- Sugar: 9.7
- Cholesterol: 15.8
- Protein: 2.3

205. Low Fat Banana Raisin French Toast

Serving: 2 serving(s) | Prep: 10mins | Ready in:

Ingredients

- 4 slices cinnamon raisin bread
- 2 large egg whites
- 1/4 cup skim milk
- 1/4 cup nonfat plain yogurt
- 1 1/2 tablespoons maple syrup or 1 1/2 tablespoons honey
- 1 teaspoon butter
- 1 ripe banana
- 2 teaspoons frozen orange juice concentrate

Direction

- Mash Banana coarsely with a fork.
- Stir in orange concentrate.

- Spread banana mixture over 2 slices of bread and top with the other two slices so you have two sandwiches.
- In a pie plate whisk together the egg whites and milk.
- Soak sandwiches for 20 seconds on each side.
- Transfer sandwiches to a plate.
- Stir together the yogurt and maple syrup set aside.
- Melt a 1/2 tsp butter in a nonstick skillet, low heat.
- With a spatula place the sandwiches in the pan and brown the underside, 5-7 minutes.
- Flip and slip the other 1/2 tsp of butter under the sandwiches and brown about 5-7 minutes.
- Serve with the sweetened yogurt.
- Turn and brown the other side 5-7 minutes.

Nutrition Information

- Calories: 306.9
- Total Fat: 4.6
- Saturated Fat: 1.9
- Fiber: 3.8
- Sodium: 314.9
- Sugar: 23.8
- Total Carbohydrate: 57.2
- Cholesterol: 6.3
- Protein: 11.5

206. Low Fat Blueberry Muffins

Serving: 12 muffins | Prep: 10mins | Ready in:

Ingredients

- 2 cups flour
- 3 teaspoons baking powder
- 4 packages Equal sugar substitute
- 1 teaspoon salt
- 1 dash nutmeg
- 1 egg
- 3/4 cup milk
- 2 tablespoons oil
- 1/2 cup applesauce
- 1 1/2 cups frozen blueberries

Direction

- Preheat oven 400' degrees F.
- Grease (or spray) 12 cup muffin tin.
- (Paper liners tend to stick).
- Combine dry ingredients in bowl.
- Beat together the milk, oil, and applesauce.
- Pour into the dry ingredients all at once and stir just until the flour is moistened (batter will be lumpy).
- Fold in blueberries.
- Fill greased muffin cups 3/4 full.
- Bake at 400 degrees approximately 20 minutes or until golden brown.
- Remove from the pan immediately.

Nutrition Information

- Calories: 145
- Total Fat: 3.5
- Total Carbohydrate: 25.6
- Cholesterol: 19.8
- Protein: 3.3
- Saturated Fat: 0.8
- Sodium: 301.6
- Fiber: 1.3
- Sugar: 6

207. Low Fat Bran Muffins

Serving: 36 muffins | Prep: 25mins | Ready in:

Ingredients

- 2 cups whole wheat flour
- 3 cups white flour
- 5 teaspoons baking soda
- 1 tablespoon salt (or less)
- 1 1/2 cups brown sugar

- 3 cups natural bran
- 3 cups all-bran cereal
- 2 cups raisins
- 2 eggs
- 2 egg whites
- 1 cup applesauce
- 1/4 cup molasses
- 1 quart 1% fat buttermilk
- 1 1/2 cups water

Direction

- Mix dry ingredients in a large bowl and make a well in the centre.
- Beat eggs and egg whites in a separate bowl and add all liquid ingredients.
- Add to dry mixture and mix well.
- Refrigerate overnight.
- Preheat oven to 400°.
- Stir batter well and fill regular muffin tins 2/3 full.
- Bake for 17-20 minutes.
- Batter will keep well in fridge at least one week.

Nutrition Information

- Calories: 173.3
- Total Fat: 1.3
- Fiber: 4.4
- Sugar: 17.9
- Total Carbohydrate: 40
- Cholesterol: 12.8
- Protein: 5
- Saturated Fat: 0.3
- Sodium: 436.4

208. Low Fat Cheesy Spinach And Egg Muffins

Serving: 12 muffins, 6 serving(s) | Prep: 10mins | Ready in:

Ingredients

- 18 slices deli turkey
- 12 large egg whites
- 1/2 cup salsa
- 1/4 cup mexican cheese
- 2 cups fresh spinach or 5 ounces frozen spinach
- 2 tablespoons Molly McButter (optional)

Direction

- Preheat oven to 350 degrees. Spray regular sized muffin tin or use foil liners. Recipe makes 12 regular muffins filled all the way to the top or 24 mini muffins. Chop turkey and spinach or use food processor. I prefer larger pieces so I use a knife. Separate egg whites into bowl saving egg yolks for Cheesy Bacon Egg Muffins (for DH and kids) Mix all ingredients together and pour into muffin tin. Bake at least 20 minutes at 350 degrees for moist squishy muffins or up to 30 minutes for a dryer more solid texture.

Nutrition Information

- Calories: 158.2
- Fiber: 0.9
- Protein: 20.5
- Total Fat: 4.4
- Saturated Fat: 1.2
- Sodium: 1329.8
- Sugar: 4.8
- Total Carbohydrate: 9
- Cholesterol: 52.6

209. Low Fat Mini Apple Crumble Muffins

Serving: 22 mini muffins, 22 serving(s) | Prep: 10mins | Ready in:

Ingredients

- 1 cup wholemeal self-rising flour

- 2 tablespoons sugar substitute
- 1/2 teaspoon cinnamon
- 2 tablespoons oil
- 1/2 cup skim milk
- 1 apple, peeled and chopped into small pieces
- 2 tablespoons oats

Direction

- Heat oven at 200 degrees Celsius, and spray mini muffin tins.
- Mix in a large bowl, flour, sugar substitute, cinnamon.
- Stir in oil, milk and apples, mix gentle to make sure all flour has been incorporated. Do not overstir.
- Place 1/2 tablespoons into mini muffin tin to just come up 3/4 of the tins.
- Sprinkle a few oats on top and place in oven.
- Bake for 10-15 minutes until brown and springs back when touched.
- Enjoy when fresh out of oven!

Nutrition Information

- Calories: 23.6
- Cholesterol: 0.1
- Sugar: 1.4
- Sodium: 3.4
- Fiber: 0.3
- Total Carbohydrate: 2.7
- Protein: 0.4
- Total Fat: 1.3
- Saturated Fat: 0.2

210. Low Fat Oatmeal Pumpkin Spice Muffins

Serving: 12 serving(s) | Prep: 10mins | Ready in:

Ingredients

- 1 1/4 cups flour
- 3/4 cup sugar
- 1 teaspoon salt
- 1 teaspoon baking powder
- 1/2 teaspoon baking soda
- 1 teaspoon cinnamon
- 1/2 teaspoon nutmeg
- 1 cup oats
- 1 1/4 cups pumpkin puree
- 1/4 cup oil
- 2 eggs, beaten
- 1/2 cup milk

Direction

- Preheat oven to 350.
- Oil or spray muffin tins with cooking spray.
- Sift together the dry ingredients.
- Add the rest of the ingredients and stir until just moistened.
- Divide into 12 muffins and bake for 15-20 minutes until cooked in center.
- Remove from pan after 5-10 minutes and let cool.
- Place in an airtight container and try not to eat for 24 hours as they will become moister.

Nutrition Information

- Calories: 209.3
- Protein: 5.1
- Sodium: 294.1
- Fiber: 1.9
- Sugar: 12.7
- Cholesterol: 32.4
- Total Fat: 6.8
- Saturated Fat: 1.3
- Total Carbohydrate: 32.7

211. Low Fat Oaty Apple Raspberry Muffins

Serving: 10 muffins, 10 serving(s) | Prep: 5mins | Ready in:

Ingredients

- 1 1/2 cups self raising flour, wholemeal
- 2 tablespoons butter, melted
- 1/2 cup skim milk
- 1/2 cup rolled oats
- 400 g apple pie filling, chopped roughly
- 3/4 cup frozen raspberries
- 1 egg
- 1 tablespoon raw sugar

Direction

- Mix flour, sugar, and oats in bowl.
- Mix melted butter, lightly beaten egg and milk in another bowl.
- Add chopped up apple and raspberry then pour all into dry ingredients.
- Mix lightly until ingredients are barely wet.
- Put into small muffin pan.
- Bake in 180 degree oven for 15-20 minutes or until cooked.

Nutrition Information

- Calories: 181.2
- Saturated Fat: 1.7
- Sodium: 48.9
- Protein: 3.9
- Total Fat: 3.3
- Fiber: 2.1
- Sugar: 11
- Total Carbohydrate: 34.4
- Cholesterol: 27.5

212. Low Fat Yogurt Biscuits

Serving: 8 biscuits | Prep: 10mins | Ready in:

Ingredients

- 1 1/2 cups all-purpose flour
- 1/2 cup whole wheat pastry flour
- 2 teaspoons baking powder
- 1/2 teaspoon salt
- 2 tablespoons vegetable oil
- 1 cup nonfat plain yogurt

Direction

- Preheat oven to 400.
- Combine all-purpose and pastry flour with baking powder and salt.
- In a separate bowl, combine yogurt and oil.
- Blend yogurt mixture into flour mixture just until the dry ingredients are moistened and it forms a dough.
- On a floured surface, pat the dough out into a circle 3/4-inch thick.
- Using a knife or a pizza cutter, cut the circle into eight wedges.
- Place wedges on an oiled baking sheet or a baking stone.
- Bake for 20 minutes or until a knife inserted in the center comes out clean.

Nutrition Information

- Calories: 158.5
- Sugar: 2.5
- Cholesterol: 0.6
- Total Fat: 3.8
- Saturated Fat: 0.5
- Sodium: 260.5
- Protein: 5.2
- Fiber: 1.6
- Total Carbohydrate: 26

213. Low Low Fat Best Blueberry Muffins

Serving: 12 muffins, 12 serving(s) | Prep: 15mins | Ready in:

Ingredients

- 1 cup dry oatmeal
- 1 cup skim milk
- 1/2 cup plain yogurt or 1/2 cup applesauce
- 1/2 cup sugar

- 1 teaspoon vanilla extract
- 1 egg
- 1/2 cup whole wheat flour
- 1/2 cup all-purpose flour
- 1 teaspoon baking powder
- 1 teaspoon baking soda
- 1/4 teaspoon salt
- 1/2 cup blueberries

Direction

- Preheat oven to 375 degrees -- spray muffin pan.
- Combine oats and milk in a small bowl, let sit.
- Sift together the flours and all dry ingredients.
- Mix together the egg, sugar, applesauce/yogurt, and vanilla.
- Mix in the oats mixture into the egg mixture.
- Fold in the dry ingredients.
- Fold in blueberries
- Transfer into pan.
- Bake 15-20 minutes for muffin tin.
- Take out, ENJOY!

Nutrition Information

- Calories: 119.5
- Fiber: 1.6
- Sugar: 9.6
- Total Carbohydrate: 23.1
- Protein: 4
- Saturated Fat: 0.5
- Sodium: 206.9
- Cholesterol: 19.4
- Total Fat: 1.4

214. Low Cal Banana Bread

Serving: 12 serving(s) | Prep: 10mins | Ready in:

Ingredients

- 1/2 cup brown sugar
- 1/4 cup margarine

- 3 eggs
- 2 2/3 cups flour
- 1 1/2 teaspoons baking powder
- 1/2 teaspoon baking soda
- 1 teaspoon salt
- 4 ripe bananas, mashed
- 1/4 cup chopped walnuts

Direction

- Preheat oven to 350 deg. F.
- Cream margarine and sugar together.
- Add eggs, one at a time, beating well after each.
- Sift dry ingredients together.
- Add bananas and dry ingredients alternately into egg mixture.
- Stir in chopped nuts.
- Pour into greased or lined loaf pans.
- Bake 20-30 minutes in small pans, 40-60 minutes in large pan until knife comes out clean.

Nutrition Information

- Calories: 239.1
- Total Fat: 7
- Fiber: 1.9
- Saturated Fat: 1.3
- Sodium: 358
- Sugar: 13.9
- Total Carbohydrate: 39.7
- Cholesterol: 52.9
- Protein: 5.3

215. Low Fat Apple Orange Oat Bran Muffins

Serving: 24-14 muffins | Prep: 10mins | Ready in:

Ingredients

- 1 1/2 cups oat bran
- 1/2 cup whole wheat flour

- 1/4 cup packed brown sugar
- 1 1/2 teaspoons baking powder
- 1 teaspoon baking soda
- 1/2 teaspoon cinnamon
- 1/2 teaspoon salt
- 1 cup buttermilk
- 1 egg
- 1 tablespoon grated orange rind
- 2 tablespoons orange juice
- 1 peeled and diced apple
- 1 cup raisins

Direction

- In large bowl, combine flour, sugar, oat bran, baking powder and soda, salt and cinnamon.
- Combine buttermilk, egg, orange rind and juice in a separate bowl.
- Stir wet ingredients into dry ingredients, mixing just until moistened.
- Stir in apples and raisins.
- Spoon into greased muffin tins.
- Sprinkle with wheat germ.
- Bake at 400 for 18-20 minutes.

Nutrition Information

- Calories: 61.8
- Fiber: 1.6
- Sugar: 7.3
- Cholesterol: 8.2
- Protein: 2.2
- Total Fat: 0.8
- Sodium: 138.9
- Total Carbohydrate: 14.6
- Saturated Fat: 0.2

216. Low Fat Blueberry Scones (Using Heart Healthy Bisquick Mix)

Serving: 8 serving(s) | Prep: 10mins | Ready in:

Ingredients

- 1 1/2 cups Bisquick baking mix (I use Heart Healthy type, see note below)
- 2 tablespoons sugar
- 1 teaspoon lemon zest, if available
- 1/2 cup blueberries
- 1 egg
- 3 tablespoons milk
- Optional glaze
- 1 -2 teaspoon lemon juice
- 1/2 cup confectioners' sugar

Direction

- NOTE: I make these scones using the "Bisquick Heart Healthy" lower fat product, but the nutrition content stated is for Standard Bisquick.
- In a large bowl, gently toss Bisquick Mix, sugar and blueberries. If you have a fresh lemon, you can also add 1 t. lemon ZEST for a great flavour boost. Set aside dry mixture.
- In a 1 cup measure, whisk milk and egg together.
- Pour liquids into Bisquick bowl and use a fork to mix things together gently. Use a large cookie scoop to portion out 8 dollops of dough onto parchment paper.
- Use wet fingers to flatten each scone slightly.
- Bake 400 degrees for 10 minutes or until edges are browning.
- Glaze: Mix lemon juice with Confectioners' Sugar to achieve a thin consistency. Drizzle over cooled scones.
- NOTE: Due to low fat content, these probably won't freeze very well, so make them and eat them!

Nutrition Information

- Calories: 162.2
- Fiber: 0.8
- Total Carbohydrate: 27.6
- Protein: 3
- Total Fat: 4.5
- Saturated Fat: 1.3

- Sodium: 254.8
- Sugar: 14.2
- Cholesterol: 24.5

217. Low Fat High Fiber Blueberry Bran Muffins

Serving: 15 serving(s) | Prep: 10mins | Ready in:

Ingredients

- 1 1/2 cups wheat bran (I used oat bran)
- 1 cup nonfat milk
- 1/2 cup unsweetened applesauce
- 1 egg
- 2/3 cup brown sugar (I used 1/2 cup)
- 1/2 teaspoon vanilla extract
- 1/2 cup all-purpose flour
- 1/2 cup whole wheat flour
- 1 teaspoon baking soda
- 1 teaspoon baking powder
- 1/2 teaspoon salt
- 1 cup blueberries (I added a chopped apple.)

Direction

- Preheat oven to 375 degrees.
- Grease muffin cups or use paper muffin liners.
- Mix together wheat bran and milk, and let stand for 10 minutes. (I didn't do this and muffins turned out fine.).
- In a large bowl, mix together applesauce, egg, brown sugar, and vanilla.
- Beat in bran mixture.
- Sift together all-purpose flour, whole wheat flour, baking soda, baking powder, and salt.
- Stir into bran mixture until just blended. Fold in blueberries.
- Scoop into muffin cups.
- Bake in preheated oven for 15 to 20 minutes, or until tops spring back when lightly tapped.

Nutrition Information

- Calories: 98.4
- Saturated Fat: 0.2
- Total Carbohydrate: 22.7
- Cholesterol: 12.7
- Protein: 2.9
- Total Fat: 0.8
- Sodium: 200.5
- Fiber: 3.4
- Sugar: 12.2

218. Low Fat Homemade Biscuits

Serving: 8-12 serving(s) | Prep: 10mins | Ready in:

Ingredients

- 2 cups whole wheat flour
- 4 teaspoons baking powder
- 3/4 teaspoon salt
- 2 tablespoons honey (add more if you want a sweeter biscuit)
- 1/3 cup vanilla yogurt
- 3/4 cup milk

Direction

- Preheat oven to 425 degrees.
- In a bowl, combine flour, baking powder, and salt.
- Add yogurt and honey. With a fork, "cut in" the yogurt and honey to the dry ingredients (like you would with butter), and combine until crumbly.
- Add milk and stir until the dough forms a ball.
- Pat or roll the dough out to 1/2-1 inch thick (depending on how big you want your biscuits).
- With a floured glass or circular cutter, cut dough into circles.
- Place biscuits on a greased cookie sheet.
- Bake for 10-12 minutes, or until lightly browned on top.

- Enjoy with honey, butter, gravy, cheese or plain!
- *** Another version of this biscuit (we call it "The Breakfast Version") ***.
- Add 1/2-3/4 cup of raisins
- 1 tablespoon cinnamon.
- Serve with applesauce.

Nutrition Information

- Calories: 139.7
- Total Fat: 1.7
- Saturated Fat: 0.8
- Sugar: 4.9
- Sodium: 417.2
- Fiber: 3.7
- Total Carbohydrate: 28.2
- Cholesterol: 4.5
- Protein: 5.2

219. Low Fat Oatmeal Pumpkin Muffins

Serving: 12 muffins, 12 serving(s) | Prep: 5mins | Ready in:

Ingredients

- 1 1/2 cups all-purpose flour
- 1 cup quick oats
- 3/4 cup firmly packed brown sugar
- 1 teaspoon baking powder
- 1/2 teaspoon baking soda
- 1 1/2 teaspoons pumpkin pie spice
- 1 cup canned pumpkin
- 3/4 cup nonfat milk
- 1/3 cup unsweetened applesauce
- 2 egg whites
- 1/4 teaspoon vanilla extract

Direction

- Preheat to 400.
- Whisk the dry ingredients together.
- Wisk wet ingredients together.
- Combine the wet and the dry.
- Grease muffin cups or tins.
- Bake for 22-25 minutes and enjoy!

Nutrition Information

- Calories: 153.9
- Sodium: 155.2
- Sugar: 14.9
- Total Carbohydrate: 33.3
- Protein: 4.1
- Total Fat: 0.7
- Saturated Fat: 0.2
- Fiber: 1.8
- Cholesterol: 0.3

220. Low Fat, High Fiber Orange Bran Muffins

Serving: 12 serving(s) | Prep: 7mins | Ready in:

Ingredients

- 1 orange, with peel, cut up
- 1/2 cup orange juice
- 1 egg
- 1/4 cup butter
- 1/4 cup unsweetened applesauce
- 1 1/4 cups flour
- 1/2 cup natural bran
- 1/2 cup white sugar
- 1 teaspoon baking powder
- 1 teaspoon baking soda
- 1/2 cup blueberries

Direction

- Cut orange into pieces, remove seeds; leave peel on.
- Put in blender and puree along with orange juice.
- Add egg, butter and applesauce.
- Puree again.

- Combine dry ingredients, stir in contents of blender.
- Barely mix in blueberries.
- Spoon muffin cups 3/4 full.
- Bake at 375 for 17 minutes.

Nutrition Information

- Calories: 141.8
- Saturated Fat: 2.6
- Protein: 2.5
- Cholesterol: 27.8
- Total Fat: 4.6
- Sodium: 174.8
- Fiber: 1.6
- Sugar: 11.3
- Total Carbohydrate: 24.1

221. Lower Fat Lemon Blueberry Scones

Serving: 16 scones, 8 serving(s) | Prep: 15mins | Ready in:

Ingredients

- For Scones
- 2 lemons
- 1 cup unbleached bread flour
- 1 cup whole wheat flour
- 1/3 cup sugar
- 2 1/2 teaspoons baking powder
- 1/2 teaspoon salt
- 3 tablespoons unsalted butter
- 2 tablespoons low-fat cream cheese
- 1 large egg, beaten
- 1 teaspoon vanilla
- 1/4 cup buttermilk
- 1/4 cup blueberries
- For Lemon Drizzle
- 1 cup powdered sugar
- 1/4 teaspoon salt

Direction

- For Scones:
- Preheat oven to 400 F and cover a cookie sheet with parchment.
- Zest the two lemons and set aside, then juice both lemons and place in a separate bowl. You'll be using the juice in both the scones and the drizzle.
- Cut up butter into small pieces, and place in freezer while completing the rest of the steps.
- Put both flours, sugar, baking powder, salt, and lemon zest in the bowl of a food processor, and process until mixed.
- In a small bowl, beat egg, vanilla, and buttermilk together. Set aside.
- Add cream cheese and butter to the dry ingredients in the food processor. Pulse until the mixture forms large crumbs.
- Add one tablespoon of reserved lemon juice (save the remaining juice for the drizzle) to the mixture in the food processor and pulse a few times.
- While pulsing the processor, add the egg, vanilla and buttermilk mixture to the rest of the mix in a slow steady stream. Continue to mix until it all holds together. The dough is a bit softer than some scone recipes. It may stick a bit, but don't be alarmed.
- Flour your counter top liberally, and dump dough out. Gently toss the dough in the flour to make it easier to work with.
- Gently knead in the blueberries (I use frozen and keep them frozen right up until this step), being careful not to overwork the dough.
- Half the dough, and press each into a small circle. Then cut each circle into eight wedges. Place the wedges on the cookie sheet.
- If you wish (and I do) sprinkle each scone with a bit of sugar.
- Bake for 15 minutes or until lightly golden.
- For Lemon Drizzle:
- Place powdered sugar and salt into a small bowl and mix well.
- Add the remaining lemon juice from the scone recipe one tablespoon at a time, and mix well until a loose glaze forms.

- To serve, pour drizzle over each scone and enjoy!

Nutrition Information

- Calories: 271.6
- Cholesterol: 37.6
- Sodium: 362.2
- Fiber: 2.5
- Sugar: 24.5
- Total Carbohydrate: 49.5
- Protein: 5.6
- Total Fat: 6.5
- Saturated Fat: 3.5

222. Lower Fat Raisin Bran Muffins

Serving: 12 muffins, 12 serving(s) | Prep: 10mins | Ready in:

Ingredients

- 2 1/2 cups Raisin Bran cereal
- 1 cup unsweetened applesauce
- 1 egg
- 1/4 cup water
- 1 cup whole wheat flour
- 2/3 cup packed brown sugar
- 1 tablespoon baking powder
- 1 1/2 teaspoons ground cinnamon

Direction

- Preheat oven to 400°F
- Spray 12 (2.5 inch) muffin cups with nonstick spray or use paper muffin cups.
- In a large bowl, stir together cereal, applesauce, egg, and water.
- Let stand 5 minutes, then stir to break up cereal.
- Add remaining ingredients; stir to combine.
- Divide evenly among muffin cups.
- Bake 15-20 minutes.

- Cool slightly, and remove from muffin cups.

Nutrition Information

- Calories: 136.2
- Sugar: 15.8
- Total Carbohydrate: 31.6
- Cholesterol: 17.6
- Total Fat: 0.9
- Sodium: 177.8
- Fiber: 3.1
- Saturated Fat: 0.2
- Protein: 3

223. Malt O Meal's Magic Muffins (Sugar Free)

Serving: 10 muffins | Prep: 10mins | Ready in:

Ingredients

- 1 1/4 cups all-purpose flour
- 3/4 cup Malt-o-Meal original hot cereal
- 1/2 cup Splenda sugar substitute
- 3/4 cup milk
- 1/4 cup vegetable oil
- 1 egg
- 1 tablespoon baking powder
- 1/2 teaspoon salt
- 1 teaspoon vanilla

Direction

- Preheat oven to 400 degrees.
- In a large mixing bowl, combine all ingredients. Stir together until all ingredients are moistened.
- Pour batter into greased or paper-lined muffin pans, filling cups 3/4 full. (I used exactly 1/4 cup for each and it made 10 muffins, not 12.).
- Bake 18-20 minutes, until center is firm to the touch.

Nutrition Information

- Calories: 157.8
- Total Fat: 6.8
- Sodium: 242.2
- Fiber: 0.7
- Total Carbohydrate: 20.5
- Protein: 3.6
- Saturated Fat: 1.3
- Sugar: 2.5
- Cholesterol: 21.2

224. Mary's Oat Bran Muffins

Serving: 12 muffins, 12 serving(s) | Prep: 10mins | Ready in:

Ingredients

- 1 1/2 cups bran flakes
- 1 1/4 cups oatmeal
- 2 1/2 cups flour
- 1 cup brown sugar (sifted)
- 4 teaspoons baking soda
- 1 teaspoon salt
- 1/2 cup vegetable oil
- 2 cups buttermilk
- 1 tablespoon molasses

Direction

- Stir all ingredients together.
- Bake at 350* about 20 minutes or until they spring back to touch.
- NOTE: This batter can be stored in the fridge for up to 2 weeks.

Nutrition Information

- Calories: 313.1
- Total Carbohydrate: 50.4
- Cholesterol: 1.6
- Total Fat: 10.3
- Saturated Fat: 1.6
- Sodium: 699.4
- Fiber: 2.4
- Sugar: 21.5
- Protein: 5.9

225. Mary's Skillet Cornbread

Serving: 4 serving(s) | Prep: 10mins | Ready in:

Ingredients

- 1 1/2 cups cornmeal
- 1/2 cup sifted flour
- 1 teaspoon baking soda
- 1 teaspoon salt
- 2 tablespoons sugar
- 1 egg
- 2 tablespoons butter
- 1 3/4 cups buttermilk

Direction

- In a mixing bowl; stir corn meal, flour, soda, salt sugar into pea size shapes.
- In a 450 degree oven in a heavy skillet heat butter till melted and sizzling but not brown.
- Meanwhile add egg and buttermilk to dry ingredients beat until completely combined.
- Stir in butter and pour into hot skillet until golden brown and bake for 20-25 minute.

Nutrition Information

- Calories: 359
- Fiber: 3.8
- Sugar: 11.9
- Cholesterol: 72.4
- Protein: 10.5
- Sodium: 1083.3
- Total Carbohydrate: 58.6
- Total Fat: 9.7
- Saturated Fat: 4.9

226. Matthew's Healthy Low Fat Vegan Carrot Spice Muffins

Serving: 12 muffins, 12 serving(s) | Prep: 5mins | Ready in:

Ingredients

- 1 3/4 cups whole wheat graham flour
- 1/4 cup sugar
- 1 tablespoon ground flax seeds
- 1 teaspoon baking powder
- 1 teaspoon baking soda
- 1 teaspoon ground cinnamon
- 3/4 teaspoon ginger
- 1/4 teaspoon pumpkin spice
- 1/2 teaspoon salt
- 2/3 cup unsweetened applesauce
- 1/2 cup vanilla soymilk
- 1/4 cup water
- 1 teaspoon vanilla
- 1 cup shredded carrot
- 1/2 cup raisins

Direction

- Mix dry ingredients in a large bowl, add the liquid ingredients and stir just long enough to combine. Add the carrots and raisins and stir to combine.
- Preheat oven to 400 degrees. Spray muffin pans with non-stick spray. Spoon the batter into the muffin cups. Bake for 15 to 20 minutes, until toothpick comes out clean.

Nutrition Information

- Calories: 104.7
- Protein: 2.7
- Total Fat: 0.9
- Saturated Fat: 0.1
- Fiber: 2.6
- Sugar: 10
- Sodium: 246.2
- Total Carbohydrate: 23.2
- Cholesterol: 0

227. Meg's Ham And Apple Biscuits

Serving: 2 serving(s) | Prep: 10mins | Ready in:

Ingredients

- 1 (16 ounce) package refrigerated biscuits (1 tube, I use the pilsbury flakey roll as they can be stretched)
- 1/2 lb thin sliced virginia ham
- 1/2 lb swiss cheese, sliced thin
- 2 apples (I use granny smiths, but any thing will do according to your taste)

Direction

- Open can of biscuits and remove biscuits.
- Take the first one and separate it into 2 halves. (I like to stretch the 2 halves a little to have more room for the filling, and it makes it easier to close them.).
- Place ham, Swiss, and apples on one half. (It doesn't matter what order they are placed in)
- Cover it with second half and seal around the edges, by pinching them together.
- Repeat with the rest of the biscuits and fillings.
- Follow baking directions according to the biscuit package.
- Bake until light brown, and enjoy.

Nutrition Information

- Calories: 1460.9
- Total Fat: 71.6
- Sodium: 4664.4
- Total Carbohydrate: 132.9
- Cholesterol: 163.3
- Protein: 71.4
- Saturated Fat: 30.8
- Fiber: 6.9
- Sugar: 34.3

228. Mexican Bizcochitos (Crusty Sweet Biscuit)

Serving: 24 biscuits | Prep: 10mins | Ready in:

Ingredients

- 1/2 cup butter
- 2 tablespoons powdered sugar
- 3/4 cup flour, plus
- 2 tablespoons flour
- 1 cup chopped pecans
- 1 teaspoon vanilla
- extra powdered sugar (in a flat dish or plate)

Direction

- Cream together butter and powdered sugar.
- Add in flour, pecans and vanilla and mix together.
- Roll dough into 1-inch balls.
- Place on a greased baking sheet.
- Flatten with bottom of a glass that has been dipped in powdered sugar.
- Bake in 300°F preheated oven for 15-20 minutes.
- When done, roll each in powdered sugar while still warm.
- If you like cinnamon, you may add it to the dough or in the powdered sugar you roll the baked biscuit inches.
- My granddaughter likes to spread a little jam on hers, but that is too sweet for me.
- Best served warm from the oven with coffee, hot chocolate or your favorite warm drink.

Nutrition Information

- Calories: 85
- Saturated Fat: 2.7
- Fiber: 0.6
- Cholesterol: 10.2
- Total Fat: 7.2
- Sodium: 27.4
- Sugar: 0.9
- Total Carbohydrate: 4.8
- Protein: 0.9

229. Mimi's Banana Muffins

Serving: 24 mini muffins | Prep: 7mins | Ready in:

Ingredients

- 2 ripe bananas
- 1/4 cup sugar
- 1/4 cup brown sugar
- 1 egg
- 1 1/4 cups whole wheat flour
- 2 teaspoons baking powder
- 1/2 teaspoon baking soda
- 4 ounces applesauce
- 1 tablespoon water
- 1 teaspoon cinnamon

Direction

- Preheat oven to 375 degrees.
- Mush bananas and combine with all the other ingredients. Spoon batter into greased muffin cups and bake for 13-15 minutes.

Nutrition Information

- Calories: 53.8
- Fiber: 1.1
- Sugar: 5.5
- Total Carbohydrate: 12.2
- Cholesterol: 8.8
- Protein: 1.2
- Sodium: 62.1
- Saturated Fat: 0.1
- Total Fat: 0.4

230. Mimi's Gingerbread Scones

Serving: 8 scones, 8 serving(s) | Prep: 15mins | Ready in:

Ingredients

- 2 cups flour
- 1/3 cup light brown sugar
- 2 teaspoons baking powder
- 1 teaspoon ginger
- 1/2 teaspoon baking soda
- 1/2 teaspoon salt
- 3/4 teaspoon ground cinnamon
- 1/8 teaspoon ground cloves
- 1/4 cup butter (room temperature)
- 1 egg
- 1 egg white
- 1/3 cup molasses (half blackstrap if you have it)
- 1/4 cup milk, plus
- 1 tablespoon milk
- 1 teaspoon vinegar
- 1 egg white (beaten and save)
- sugar, for sprinkling

Direction

- Combine the first eight ingredients.
- With a pastry blender, cut in the butter till there are coarse crumbs.
- Make a well in the center.
- In small bowl mix the next five ingredients-- the egg, egg white, molasses, milk, and vinegar.
- Mix this well; it may be a little dry.
- Put on floured board and knead a few times till smooth.
- Pat into a 7" circle and cut into 8 wedges.
- Arrange on an ungreased baking sheet having the wedges 1" apart.
- Brush with the extra beaten egg white and sprinkle with sugar.
- Bake in a 400 degree oven for 12-15 minutes.
- Cool on a wire rack for 20 minutes.
- Serve warm.

Nutrition Information

- Calories: 261.5
- Saturated Fat: 4.1
- Sodium: 392.4
- Sugar: 16.8
- Total Fat: 7.1
- Fiber: 1
- Total Carbohydrate: 44.4
- Cholesterol: 43
- Protein: 5.3

231. Mini Cinnamon Raisin Muffins

Serving: 48 Mini Muffins | Prep: 10mins | Ready in:

Ingredients

- 2 cups flour
- 1 tablespoon baking powder
- 1/2 teaspoon salt
- 1 1/2 teaspoons cinnamon
- 2 eggs
- 1 cup milk
- 2/3 cup packed brown sugar
- 6 tablespoons unsalted butter
- 1 teaspoon vanilla
- 1 cup raisins
- Topping
- 1/4 cup sugar
- 1 teaspoon cinnamon

Direction

- Preheat oven to 400.
- Spray a 24 count mini muffin pan with non-stick spray.
- Make topping in small bowl; set aside.
- In large bowl mix together flour, baking powder, salt, and cinnamon, set aside.
- In another bowl cream the butter and brown sugar until light and fluffy, about 3 minutes.
- Add eggs, one at a time, beating well after each addition.

- Beat in vanilla extract.
- Beat in dry ingredients until just incorporated.
- Stir in raisins.
- Using a small scoop, fill muffin pan, and then sprinkle each one with cinnamon sugar topping.
- Bake for 10 to 12 minutes.

Nutrition Information

- Calories: 63.3
- Sodium: 53.9
- Total Carbohydrate: 10.8
- Cholesterol: 12.3
- Protein: 1.1
- Total Fat: 1.9
- Saturated Fat: 1.1
- Fiber: 0.3
- Sugar: 5.8

232. Mini Ginger Scones

Serving: 16 mini scones, 16 serving(s) | Prep: 15mins | Ready in:

Ingredients

- 2 cups flour
- 1/4 cup sugar
- 1 1/4 teaspoons baking powder
- 1/4 teaspoon baking soda
- 1/4 teaspoon salt
- 1/2 cup butter, cold and cut into pieces
- 1/4 cup candied ginger, diced
- 1/2 teaspoon cinnamon
- 1/4 teaspoon cardamom
- 1 pinch clove
- 3/4 cup buttermilk

Direction

- Heat oven to 400°F Brush pan with vegetable shortening or butter. In a large bowl, sift together flour, sugar, baking powder, baking soda, and salt. Blend butter into the flour mixture with a pastry blender or two knives. The mixture should look like course meal. Stir in candied ginger. Add buttermilk to the flour mixture. Stir just until the dough comes together. Do not over mix the dough. Divide dough evenly among wells in pan. Bake for 13-18 minutes, until golden brown and toothpick comes out clean. Cool 10 minutes in pan. Remove from pan and serve.

Nutrition Information

- Calories: 124.9
- Fiber: 0.5
- Sugar: 3.7
- Total Carbohydrate: 15.8
- Total Fat: 6
- Saturated Fat: 3.7
- Protein: 2.1
- Sodium: 147.4
- Cholesterol: 15.7

233. Mini Holiday Muffins

Serving: 24 serving(s) | Prep: 15mins | Ready in:

Ingredients

- 1/4 cup butter
- 1/2 cup sugar
- 1/2 cup brown sugar
- 2 eggs, separated
- 1 tablespoon maraschino cherry juice
- 1 cup flour
- 1/4 teaspoon baking powder
- 24 maraschino cherries
- 1 cup pecans, finely chopped
- powdered sugar

Direction

- Cream butter and sugar together.

- Mix in beaten egg yolks, cherry juice, flour and baking powder.
- Beat egg whites until stiff and fold into mixture.
- Grease mini muffins tins and sprinkle bottom with chopped pecans.
- Place 1 teaspoon dough in each and place cherry on top.
- Add another teaspoon full of dough and sprinkle top with pecans.
- Bake at 350°F for 10 minutes.
- Remove from muffin tins and roll in powdered sugar while still warm.
- Makes 24 mini muffins.

Nutrition Information

- Calories: 115.1
- Cholesterol: 22.7
- Protein: 1.5
- Total Fat: 5.7
- Sodium: 25.3
- Fiber: 0.7
- Sugar: 10.7
- Saturated Fat: 1.6
- Total Carbohydrate: 15.4

234. Miniature Mango Muffins

Serving: 18 serving(s) | Prep: 20mins | Ready in:

Ingredients

- 1/2 cup whole wheat flour
- 1/2 cup all-purpose flour
- 2 tablespoons wheat germ
- 2 tablespoons firmly packed brown sugar
- 1/2 teaspoon baking soda
- 1/8 teaspoon salt
- 1/2 cup mashed mango
- 1 1/2 tablespoons vegetable oil
- 1 egg, beaten
- 2 1/4 teaspoons skim milk
- 1 1/2 teaspoons dark rum
- 1/4 teaspoon coconut extract
- 1/4 teaspoon almond extract
- vegetable oil cooking spray

Direction

- Combine first 6 ingredients in a large bowl; make a well in center of mixture. Combine mango, oil, egg, milk, rum and extracts; add liquid mixture to dry ingredients, stirring just until dry ingredients are moistened.
- Spoon batter into miniature muffin pans coated with cooking spray, filling ¾ full. Bake at 350 degrees for 10 to 12 minutes or until golden. Remove from pans, and let cool slightly on a wire rack.

Nutrition Information

- Calories: 51.1
- Cholesterol: 11.8
- Total Fat: 1.6
- Saturated Fat: 0.3
- Total Carbohydrate: 7.8
- Protein: 1.4
- Sodium: 56.4
- Fiber: 0.7
- Sugar: 2.2

235. Miracle Carrot Muffins

Serving: 12 muffins | Prep: 15mins | Ready in:

Ingredients

- 1 1/3 cups sugar
- 1/4 cup butter
- 1 1/4 cups shredded carrots
- 1 cup regular raisins (I like gold) or 1 cup gold raisins (I like gold)
- 1 teaspoon kosher salt
- 1 teaspoon cinnamon
- 1 teaspoon ground allspice
- 2 cups all-purpose flour

- 1 teaspoon baking powder
- 1 teaspoon baking soda

Direction

- Preheat oven to 375 degrees. Put sugar, butter, carrots, raisins, salt, spices and 1 1/3 cups water in a medium saucepan. Heat over high heat, stirring occasionally, just until mixture comes to a boil. Set aside to cool slightly.
- Whisk flour, baking powder and baking soda together in a medium bowl. Pour warm carrot mixture into dry ingredients. Stir to combine, but do not over mix.
- Spoon mixture into greased muffin cups. (I use cupcake paper holders in the muffin tin).
- Bake until browned and a toothpick inserted into a muffin comes out clean, about 15-20 minutes. Let cool on a rack.

Nutrition Information

- Calories: 238.5
- Total Fat: 4.1
- Sodium: 325.6
- Sugar: 30
- Protein: 2.7
- Saturated Fat: 2.5
- Fiber: 1.5
- Total Carbohydrate: 49.3
- Cholesterol: 10.2

236. Moist Cornbread Muffins

Serving: 24 muffins, 24 serving(s) | Prep: 1hours15mins | Ready in:

Ingredients

- 2 1/2 cups yellow cornmeal (I used stone ground whole grain medium grind)
- 2 cups pastry flour
- 2/3 cup raw sugar
- 2 teaspoons baking soda
- 1 teaspoon salt
- 3 eggs
- 2 1/2 cups buttermilk
- 1 cup olive oil

Direction

- At least one hour before you bake these, mix the cornmeal with the buttermilk and soak in the refrigerator. This can also be done the night before.
- Preheat oven to 425 and grease muffin tins.
- Beat eggs with olive oil and sugar. Add cornmeal-buttermilk mixture.
- Mix flour, baking soda and salt in a bowl. Add liquid ingredients and stir until just blended.
- Spoon into well-greased muffin tins, filling about 3/4 full.
- Bake 15 minutes or until tops are golden brown and spring back to the touch. Cool slightly before removing from pan - they are especially crumbly when hot.

Nutrition Information

- Calories: 207.6
- Saturated Fat: 1.7
- Fiber: 1.1
- Sugar: 6.9
- Total Carbohydrate: 25.5
- Cholesterol: 24.3
- Total Fat: 10.4
- Sodium: 242.4
- Protein: 3.6

237. Moist And Healthy Banana Muffins

Serving: 12 muffins, 12 serving(s) | Prep: 5mins | Ready in:

Ingredients

- 1 1/4 cups all-purpose flour

- 1 cup whole wheat flour
- 1/3 cup sugar
- 2 teaspoons baking powder
- 1/2 teaspoon baking soda
- 2 teaspoons cinnamon
- 1/2 teaspoon salt
- 1/2 cup low-fat buttermilk
- 1/3 cup vegetable oil
- 1 egg
- 3 really ripe bananas, mashed

Direction

- Preheat oven to 375 degrees F.
- Line 12 muffin tins with paper muffin cups or spray with non-stick cooking spray.
- Sift dry ingredients together.
- Add all liquid ingredients; mix, (don't over mix)
- Fill muffins tins 3/4 full.
- Bake in pre-heated oven for 15-20 minutes.

Nutrition Information

- Calories: 194.1
- Sodium: 227.6
- Fiber: 2.5
- Total Carbohydrate: 30.5
- Cholesterol: 18
- Protein: 3.9
- Saturated Fat: 1.1
- Total Fat: 7
- Sugar: 9.8

238. Mom T's Refrigerator Bran Muffins

Serving: 48 muffins, 48 serving(s) | Prep: 10mins | Ready in:

Ingredients

- 5/8 cup butter
- 3 cups sugar
- 4 eggs, beaten
- 1 quart buttermilk
- 2 cups all-bran cereal (pellet shape)
- 2 cups boiling water
- 5 cups flour
- 5 teaspoons baking soda
- 1 teaspoon salt
- 4 cups all-bran cereal (long type)
- 2 cups raisins (you may substitute blueberries, figs or dried apples)

Direction

- Cream butter and sugar.
- Add beaten eggs and buttermilk to butter mixture.
- Mix together and let stand a minute the All-Bran (pellets) and the boiling water. Set aside.
- Mix dry ingredients, flour, soda and salt. Add choice of fruit. Set aside.
- Add soaked All Bran to creamed mixture.
- Add dry ingredients to this. Add the All-Bran (long type) and stir slightly until mixed.
- Let stand in refrigerator 24 hours.
- When ready to use stir and then bake in greased muffin pan for approximately 20 minutes at 400 degrees.
- Store extra batter in airtight container in refrigerator.

Nutrition Information

- Calories: 169.3
- Sugar: 18.3
- Total Carbohydrate: 34
- Sodium: 249.5
- Fiber: 2.9
- Cholesterol: 22.7
- Protein: 3.8
- Total Fat: 3.5
- Saturated Fat: 1.8

239. Mom's Magic Muffins

Serving: 4 dozen | Prep: 15mins | Ready in:

Ingredients

- 1 (14 ounce) box Raisin Bran cereal
- 5 cups all-purpose flour
- 3 cups sugar
- 5 teaspoons baking soda
- 2 teaspoons salt
- 4 cups buttermilk
- 1 cup vegetable oil
- 4 eggs, beaten
- 1 1/2 cups dried sweetened cranberries

Direction

- Combine cereal, flour, sugar, baking soda and salt in a large bowl; mix well. Combine buttermilk, oil and eggs in a separate bowl and whisk well. Pour egg mixture into cereal mixture; stir until just blended. Fold in cranberries.
- Place in a tightly covered container in the refrigerator overnight. The batter will keep for four weeks and improves over time. Do not stir at any time after refrigerating or when preparing to bake the muffins.
- Preheat oven to 400°F Grease muffin cups. Spoon batter into prepared pan. Bake 18 minutes, or until a wooden pick inserted in the center comes out almost clean. Cool in muffin tins 10 minutes. Serve warm or remove to a wire rack to cool completely.

Nutrition Information

- Calories: 2257.7
- Protein: 39
- Fiber: 18.6
- Total Carbohydrate: 394.1
- Cholesterol: 221.3
- Total Fat: 66.2
- Saturated Fat: 10.8
- Sodium: 3656.1
- Sugar: 223.4

240. Mom's Southern Homemade Simple Biscuits

Serving: 4-6 serving(s) | Prep: 5mins | Ready in:

Ingredients

- 1 1/2 cups self-rising flour
- 1/2 cup milk
- 1 1/2-2 tablespoons vegetable oil

Direction

- Preheat oven to 425°F.
- Mix all ingredients well. If dough seems dry, add a little bit extra milk until mixes well.
- Place dough onto lightly greased cookie sheet in biscuit shapes. My mother didn't even shape them; she would just put globs of dough down and they would be irregular shapes.
- Lightly dust flour on the top of the biscuits.
- Bake for 25-30 minutes, or until golden brown.

Nutrition Information

- Calories: 230.5
- Sodium: 610.3
- Cholesterol: 4.3
- Saturated Fat: 1.4
- Sugar: 0.1
- Total Carbohydrate: 36.2
- Protein: 5.6
- Total Fat: 6.7
- Fiber: 1.3

241. Most Delicious Muffins

Serving: 15 muffins, 4-6 serving(s) | Prep: 10mins | Ready in:

Ingredients

- 1 cup whole wheat flour
- 1 cup rolled oats
- 1 cup natural bran
- 1/2 teaspoon salt
- 1/3 cup non-fat powdered milk
- 1/2 teaspoon baking soda
- 2 teaspoons baking powder
- 1 cup mashed banana
- 2 egg whites
- 3-4 tablespoons honey or 3-4 tablespoons maple syrup or 3-4 tablespoons molasses
- 2 tablespoons vegetable oil
- 1 cup orange juice
- 2 tablespoons dark rum or 2 teaspoons rum extract

Direction

- Preheat oven to 400 degrees.
- Combine dry ingredients.
- In a larger bowl, mash the banana and beat in the egg whites until mixture is frothy.
- Blend in the honey, vegetable oil (if using), orange juice and rum.
- Incorporate dry ingredients and blend just until combined.
- Lightly grease muffin tins and fill two-thirds.
- *This oil can be eliminated for completely fat-free muffins.
- Bake for 18-20 minutes.

Nutrition Information

- Calories: 466.4
- Sugar: 33.1
- Cholesterol: 2
- Total Fat: 9.8
- Saturated Fat: 1.4
- Sodium: 750.9
- Fiber: 11.7
- Total Carbohydrate: 84.6
- Protein: 15.8

242. Muffins

Serving: 4 dozen | Prep: 15mins | Ready in:

Ingredients

- 2 cups whole wheat flour
- 3 cups white flour
- 5 teaspoons baking soda
- 1 tablespoon salt
- 1 teaspoon cinnamon
- 1/2 teaspoon allspice
- 1 1/2 cups brown sugar
- 3 cups all-bran cereal
- 3 cups natural bran
- 2 eggs
- 2 egg whites
- 1 quart 1% fat buttermilk
- 1 cup unsweetened applesauce
- 1/4 cup molasses
- 1 1/4 cups water
- 2 cups raisins (or craisins)
- 4 cups grated carrots

Direction

- Mix together dry ingredients, set aside.
- Beat eggs and all liquid ingredients, mix well.
- Add liquid ingredients, raisins and carrots to dry mixture.
- Stir well.
- Refrigerate overnight or for at least 6 hours.
- Before baking stir the batter well.
- Preheat oven to 400.
- Fill muffin tins 1/2 full.
- Bake 17-20 minutes.
- Hints---------------.
- Do not use muffin liners- the muffins will stick to the paper really bad.
- This happens because there is no fat in the recipe.
- You must refrigerate the batter for at least 6 hours or the muffins are dry.
- You have to let the cereal soak up all the wet ingredients otherwise it stays dry.
- Enjoy!

Nutrition Information

- Calories: 1601.1
- Saturated Fat: 3.2
- Sodium: 4013.1
- Protein: 46.5
- Total Fat: 12.3
- Fiber: 43.5
- Sugar: 173.5
- Total Carbohydrate: 369.7
- Cholesterol: 102.8

243. Multi Grain Banana Muffins

Serving: 9 Muffins | Prep: 10mins | Ready in:

Ingredients

- 3 bananas
- 1/4 cup Splenda sugar substitute
- 1 egg
- 1/3 cup butter
- 1 teaspoon baking soda
- 1 teaspoon baking powder
- 1/2 teaspoon salt
- 1 1/2 cups multi-grain flour
- 1/4 cup chocolate chips

Direction

- Mash bananas. Add Splenda and egg. Add melted butter. Add dry ingredients. Stir in chocolate chips and bake at 375 for 20 minutes.

Nutrition Information

- Calories: 126
- Fiber: 1.3
- Total Carbohydrate: 12.1
- Cholesterol: 41.6
- Total Fat: 8.9
- Saturated Fat: 5.4
- Sodium: 366.4
- Sugar: 7.4
- Protein: 1.4

244. Mushroom Egg Muffin

Serving: 6 6 muffins, 1 serving(s) | Prep: 5mins | Ready in:

Ingredients

- 6 eggs
- 1/3 cup milk
- 6 teaspoons parmesan cheese
- 16 shiitake mushrooms
- 1 tablespoon olive oil
- salt, pepper
- scallion, chives (optional)

Direction

- .Wisk eggs with milk; sauté mushrooms in olive oil. Spoon mushroom to muffin tins and add egg mixture to 3/4 full. Bake 15 min at 400°F.

Nutrition Information

- Calories: 746.8
- Total Carbohydrate: 27
- Cholesterol: 1136.2
- Saturated Fat: 14.8
- Fiber: 7.6
- Protein: 51
- Total Fat: 49.4
- Sodium: 646.3
- Sugar: 8.4

245. My Favorite Muffins

Serving: 12 serving(s) | Prep: 10mins | Ready in:

Ingredients

- 1/2 pint blueberries
- 1/4 cup sugar substitute (like Splenda)
- 1 cup oatmeal
- 1 cup low-fat buttermilk
- 1/3 cup applesauce (none of that sugar-added stuff (just apples and water!)
- 1/2 cup light brown sugar
- 1/4 cup egg substitute
- 1 cup whole wheat flour
- 1 teaspoon baking powder
- 1/2 teaspoon baking soda
- 1/4 teaspoon maple extract

Direction

- Preheat oven to 400 degrees.
- Line muffin tin with paper cups.
- Mix everything except blueberries in large bowl.
- Carefully stir in blueberries.
- Spoon into muffin tins.
- Bake for about 18 minutes.

Nutrition Information

- Calories: 130.6
- Sodium: 119.4
- Sugar: 14.2
- Cholesterol: 0.8
- Saturated Fat: 0.2
- Fiber: 2.1
- Total Carbohydrate: 28.3
- Protein: 3.6
- Total Fat: 0.9

246. Nana Walnut Muffins

Serving: 16 mini muffins, 16 serving(s) | Prep: 10mins | Ready in:

Ingredients

- 1 1/3 cups whole wheat flour
- 1/2 cup Splenda granular
- 1 teaspoon baking powder
- 1 pinch kosher salt
- 1 tablespoon canola oil
- 1/3 cup nonfat milk
- 2 teaspoons vanilla
- 3 bananas
- 1/4 cup walnuts, chopped
- 1 cup oatmeal

Direction

- Preheat oven to 350 degrees. Spay mini muffin tins or use foil liners. Blend dry ingredients and set aside. Add oil, milk, and vanilla to mashed bananas. Stir in dry ingredients. And add nuts. Use ice cream scoop to put in mini pan(s). Bake until brown and toothpick test center.

Nutrition Information

- Calories: 96
- Total Carbohydrate: 16.3
- Total Fat: 2.7
- Fiber: 2.3
- Sugar: 3.2
- Cholesterol: 0.1
- Protein: 2.7
- Saturated Fat: 0.3
- Sodium: 34.7

247. Nana's Walnut Biscuits

Serving: 20 biscuits | Prep: 15mins | Ready in:

Ingredients

- 125 g butter
- 1 cup flour
- 1 egg
- 1/2 cup walnuts
- 1/2 cup sugar
- 1/2 teaspoon baking powder
- 1 tablespoon cocoa

- 1/4 cup coconut (optional)

Direction

- Cream butter and sugar, add egg and beat.
- Add sifted cocoa, flour, baking powder then nuts.
- Put teaspoon amounts onto cold greased tray, cook in medium oven.

Nutrition Information

- Calories: 110.5
- Total Fat: 7.3
- Protein: 1.5
- Saturated Fat: 3.5
- Sodium: 48.5
- Fiber: 0.4
- Sugar: 5.1
- Total Carbohydrate: 10.4
- Cholesterol: 23.9

248. New England Blueberry Muffins

Serving: 18 small muffins | Prep: 15mins | Ready in:

Ingredients

- 2 1/2 cups flour
- 1/2 cup sugar
- 3 teaspoons baking powder
- 1/2 teaspoon salt
- 2 eggs, well beaten
- 3 tablespoons butter, melted
- 1 cup milk
- 1 1/2 cups blueberries, washed and stemmed

Direction

- Preheat oven to 375F and grease muffin pans very well or line with cupcake papers.
- Sift dry ingredients together.
- Mix berries with a fourth of this mixture.
- Beat eggs; add melted butter and milk.
- Pour into dry ingredients and stir until there are no large lumps.
- Fold blueberries in lightly.
- Pour batter into prepared pans and bake for 15 to 25 minutes, depending on the size of the muffins.

Nutrition Information

- Calories: 125.7
- Protein: 3
- Total Fat: 3.1
- Fiber: 0.8
- Total Carbohydrate: 21.4
- Cholesterol: 27.6
- Saturated Fat: 1.7
- Sodium: 157.1
- Sugar: 6.8

249. Non Fat Banana Muffins

Serving: 12 muffins, 12 serving(s) | Prep: 6mins | Ready in:

Ingredients

- 1 1/2 cups all-purpose flour
- 1/2 teaspoon baking soda
- 1/2 teaspoon salt
- 1/4 teaspoon baking powder
- 1/4 teaspoon cinnamon
- 1/4 teaspoon nutmeg
- 3/4 cup sugar
- 1/4 cup honey
- 3/4 cup unsweetened applesauce
- 1/8 cup water, lukewarm
- 1/2 tablespoon vanilla extract
- 1 banana, mashed

Direction

- Preheat oven to 350 degrees Fahrenheit and line 12 muffin cups.

- Whisk flour, baking soda, salt, baking powder, cinnamon, and nutmeg in a medium bowl.
- Beat the rest and stir in bananas. Add dry ingredients and stir.
- Divide the batter among 12 muffin cups and bake on middle rack for approximately 15 minutes or until light, light brown in color.
- Let cool out of pan for a couple minutes before serving.

Nutrition Information

- Calories: 144
- Total Fat: 0.2
- Total Carbohydrate: 34.4
- Cholesterol: 0
- Protein: 1.8
- Saturated Fat: 0.1
- Sodium: 158
- Fiber: 0.9
- Sugar: 19.6

250. Oat Biscuits

Serving: 30 biscuits | Prep: 20mins | Ready in:

Ingredients

- 2 cups old fashioned oats
- 2 cups whole wheat flour
- 1 cup unsalted butter, cold, cut into pieces
- 1/3 cup dark brown sugar, packed
- 1 3/4 teaspoons baking powder
- 1 1/2 teaspoons salt
- 1/2 cup whole milk

Direction

- Coarsely chop the oats in a food processor and transfer to a large bowl. Pulse together the flour, butter, brown sugar, baking powder and salt in the food processor until mixture resembles a coarse meal. Add milk and blend until mixture just forms a dough. Add the oats and knead until just incorporated.
- Halve the dough and pat each half into a 5 by 3-inch rectangle. Chill, wrapped well in plastic wrap, until firm, about 3 hours.
- Preheat the oven to 350°F.
- Cut 1 rectangle cross-wise into scant 1/4 inch thick slices and bake on an ungreased large baking sheet in the middle of the oven until undersides are a shade darker, about 20 minutes. Transfer to a rack to cool and make more biscuits with the remaining rectangle of dough.

Nutrition Information

- Calories: 113.9
- Protein: 2.2
- Saturated Fat: 4
- Sodium: 141.5
- Fiber: 1.5
- Total Carbohydrate: 12.1
- Cholesterol: 16.7
- Total Fat: 6.8
- Sugar: 2.7

251. Oat Bran Applesauce Muffins

Serving: 24 muffins | Prep: 25mins | Ready in:

Ingredients

- 3 cups oat bran
- 2 cups whole wheat flour
- 1 cup unbleached flour
- 1 tablespoon baking powder
- 1 tablespoon baking soda
- 1 teaspoon salt
- 2 cups applesauce, chilled
- 1/2 cup olive oil or 1/2 cup vegetable oil
- 4 eggs, beaten with a fork
- 1 cup honey

Direction

- Stir together dry ingredients.
- Mix in remaining ingredients, stirring until completely combined (don't overmix them, though).
- Spoon batter into 24 greased muffin cups, and let stand 10 minutes.
- Bake muffins 15 minutes at 400 degrees, or until they are golden brown and test done; remove from pans and cool on rack.

Nutrition Information

- Calories: 193.2
- Sodium: 318.2
- Fiber: 3.5
- Sugar: 11.9
- Protein: 5.1
- Total Fat: 6.4
- Saturated Fat: 1.1
- Total Carbohydrate: 35.1
- Cholesterol: 35.2

252. Oat Bran Blueberry Mini Muffins

Serving: 24 serving(s) | Prep: 10mins | Ready in:

Ingredients

- 1 1/2 cups oat bran
- 1 cup whole wheat flour
- 2 tablespoons ground flax seeds
- 1 1/4 teaspoons baking soda
- 1 teaspoon ground cinnamon
- 1/8 teaspoon salt
- 3/4 cup skim milk
- 1/3 cup honey
- 1 medium banana, mashed
- 1 large egg
- 2 tablespoons olive oil
- 1 teaspoon vanilla extract
- 1 cup fresh blueberries

Direction

- Position a rack in the center of the oven and preheat oven to 400 degrees Fahrenheit. Lightly coat 24 nonstick miniature muffin cups with cooking oil spray.
- In a medium bowl, combine bran, flour, flaxseed, baking soda, cinnamon, and salt. Set aside. In another medium bowl or in a blender, combine the milk, honey, banana, egg, olive oil, and vanilla extract until smooth.
- Make a well in the center of the dry ingredients, and pour in one-third of the liquid mixture. Using a spoon, stir until smooth. Add remaining liquid mixture and stir just until combined. Add blueberries and stir again, but do not over mix.
- Spoon 2 tablespoons of batter into each prepared muffin cup. Bake about 8 minutes, or until the tops spring back when pressed gently in the centers. Do not overbake. Cool in the pan on a wire rack for 10 minutes before removing from the cups. Serve warm or cool completely on the rack.

Nutrition Information

- Calories: 73.5
- Cholesterol: 9
- Protein: 2.5
- Total Fat: 2.1
- Saturated Fat: 0.4
- Sodium: 86.1
- Total Carbohydrate: 14.1
- Fiber: 2
- Sugar: 5.2

253. Oat Bran Dinner Muffins

Serving: 12 muffins, 12 serving(s) | Prep: 15mins | Ready in:

Ingredients

- 1 1/4 cups oat bran
- 1 cup self-rising flour
- 1 1/2 cups evaporated skim milk
- 2 egg whites
- 2 tablespoons honey
- 3 tablespoons vegetable oil

Direction

- Preheat the oven to 425 °F. Mix the dry ingredients in a large bowl. Mix the milk and the remaining ingredients in a blender at low speed, then add to the dry ingredients and stir until just mixed.
- Line a muffin pan with paper baking cups and fill with batter.
- Bake 15 minutes or till toothpick comes out dry.

Nutrition Information

- Calories: 129.5
- Total Fat: 4.3
- Saturated Fat: 0.6
- Sodium: 178.8
- Sugar: 6.7
- Total Carbohydrate: 20.8
- Cholesterol: 1.3
- Fiber: 1.8
- Protein: 5.8

254. Oat Bran Muffins (And Variations)

Serving: 12 serving(s) | Prep: 15mins | Ready in:

Ingredients

- 2 1/4 cups unprocessed oat bran
- 1/4 cup firmly packed brown sugar
- 1 teaspoon baking powder
- 1/4 teaspoon salt
- 3/4 cup skim milk
- 1/2 cup egg substitute
- 1/4 cup honey
- 2 teaspoons vegetable oil or 2 teaspoons canola oil
- vegetable oil cooking spray

Direction

- Combine first 4 ingredients in a large bowl; make a well in the center of mixture. Combine milk, egg substitute, honey, and oil; add to dry mixture, stirring just until moistened.
- Spoon batter into muffin pans coated with cooking spray, filling three-fourths full.
- Bake at 425* for 15 minutes. Yield: 1 dozen (121 calories per muffin).
- RAISIN OAT BRAN MUFFINS: Add 1/3 cup raisins to batter.
- BANANA OAT BRAN MUFFINS: Add ½ cup mashed ripe bananas to batter.
- BLUEBERRY OAT BRAN MUFFINS: Add ½ cup fresh or frozen (thawed) Blueberries to batter.
- APPLE-CINNAMON OAT BRAN: Add ½ cup minced apple and 1 teaspoons Ground cinnamon to batter.
- CRANBERRY OAT BRAN MUFFINS: Add ¾ cup fresh or frozen (thawed) Cranberries to batter.

Nutrition Information

- Calories: 104
- Total Carbohydrate: 23
- Protein: 4.9
- Total Fat: 2.4
- Sodium: 109.1
- Fiber: 2.7
- Saturated Fat: 0.4
- Sugar: 10.5
- Cholesterol: 0.4

255. Oatmeal Banana Muffins

Serving: 18 muffins | Prep: 10mins | Ready in:

Ingredients

- 1/2 cup margarine, softened
- 1/2 cup sugar
- 2 eggs
- 1 cup mashed ripe banana
- 3/4 cup honey
- 1 1/2 cups flour
- 1 cup quick-cooking oats
- 1 teaspoon baking powder
- 1 teaspoon baking soda
- 3/4 teaspoon salt

Direction

- Cream margarine and sugar in mixing bowl.
- Add eggs, bananas and honey; mix well.
- In separate bowl, combine dry ingredients; stir into creamed mixture just until moistened.
- Line muffin tins with paper cups or grease tins.
- Fill cups 2/3 full.
- Bake in preheated 350 degree oven for 18-20 minutes.
- Cool in pan 10 minutes before removing to wire rack.

Nutrition Information

- Calories: 180.4
- Sugar: 18.3
- Total Fat: 6
- Sodium: 254.9
- Fiber: 1
- Total Carbohydrate: 30.2
- Cholesterol: 23.5
- Protein: 2.7
- Saturated Fat: 1.1

256. Oatmeal Breakfast Muffins

Serving: 12 serving(s) | Prep: 10mins | Ready in:

Ingredients

- 1 cup flour
- 1 cup whole wheat flour
- 1 cup quick-cooking oatmeal
- 1/2 teaspoon ground cinnamon
- 1/4 teaspoon ground nutmeg
- 3 teaspoons baking powder
- 1/2 teaspoon salt
- 1 cup apple juice
- 2 egg whites
- 1 egg yolk
- 1/4 cup corn oil

Direction

- Combine dry ingredients. Stir in combined remaining ingredients, stirring until just blended.
- Pour into greased muffin tins and bake at 400 for 15-20 minutes.

Nutrition Information

- Calories: 155.2
- Saturated Fat: 0.9
- Sodium: 199.1
- Fiber: 2.1
- Sugar: 2.2
- Total Fat: 5.7
- Total Carbohydrate: 22.5
- Cholesterol: 13.8
- Protein: 4.1

257. Oatmeal Cranberry Scones

Serving: 8 scones, 4 serving(s) | Prep: 10mins | Ready in:

Ingredients

- 1 1/2 cups all-purpose flour
- 1/4 cup sugar
- 1 tablespoon baking powder

- 1/2 teaspoon salt
- 1 1/4 cups rolled oats
- 1/2 cup dried cranberries (or raisins)
- 1 large egg
- 10 tablespoons unsalted butter (melted)
- 1/3 cup milk

Direction

- Preheat the oven to 450°F (230°C).
- Whisk together the flour, sugar, baking powder and salt. Stir in the oatmeal and cranberries. You may need to use your fingers to be sure the cranberries are all separated.
- Whisk together the egg, butter and milk then add the mixture to the dry ingredients. Mix together just until the dry ingredients are moistened. The dough will be sticky.
- Transfer the dough onto an ungreased baking sheet and pat into a circle about 3/4 inches (2 cm) thick. Sprinkle liberally with sugar and score the top into eight wedges.
- Bake on a rack in the middle of the oven for about 12 minutes until lightly browned.

Nutrition Information

- Calories: 609.3
- Saturated Fat: 19.4
- Cholesterol: 132
- Sodium: 596.5
- Fiber: 4.3
- Sugar: 13.6
- Total Carbohydrate: 68.6
- Protein: 11.5
- Total Fat: 32.9

258. Oatmeal Drop Biscuits

Serving: 9 Biscuits | Prep: 5mins | Ready in:

Ingredients

- 2 cups Bisquick
- 1/4 cup quick-cooking oats
- 2/3 cup skim milk

Direction

- Preheat oven to 450.
- Mix all ingredients together till moist.
- Drop by large spoonfuls onto ungreased baking sheet.
- Bake for 9-12 minutes or until tops brown.

Nutrition Information

- Calories: 130.2
- Saturated Fat: 1.1
- Fiber: 0.8
- Sugar: 3.1
- Total Carbohydrate: 19.4
- Sodium: 351.1
- Cholesterol: 0.9
- Protein: 3.2
- Total Fat: 4.3

259. Oatmeal Peanut Butter And Jelly Muffins

Serving: 12 serving(s) | Prep: 10mins | Ready in:

Ingredients

- 1 cup water
- 1/2 cup oatmeal
- 3/4 cup peanut butter (crunchy or smooth)
- 1 teaspoon vanilla
- 2/3 cup honey (or other liquid sweetener)
- 1 cup soymilk (or other nondairy milk, or cow's milk if not vegan)
- 1 cup whole wheat flour
- 1 cup unbleached white flour
- 1/2 cup barley flour
- 1 teaspoon baking soda
- 1 teaspoon baking powder
- 1/2 teaspoon salt

- 9 ounces raspberry preserves (or favorite flavor jelly or jam)

Direction

- Preheat the oven to 350 degrees F. Lightly oil 12-cup muffin tin.
- In a 2 cup bowl, combine water and oatmeal and microwave for 5 minutes or until cooked. (Alternatively, use 1 cup leftover oatmeal).
- In a medium mixing bowl, mix the cooked oatmeal with the peanut butter, vanilla, honey, and milk. Stir until all the lumps are gone.
- In another bowl, combine the flours, baking soda, baking powder, and salt. Add the dry ingredients to the liquid ingredients, and stir well. Fill muffin tins evenly with batter and bake for 20 minutes.
- Test to see if the muffins are done by inserting a toothpick in the middle of a muffin. If the toothpick comes out clean, the muffins are done. Remove from tins and place on a solid surface.
- Spoon preserves into a pastry bag fitted with whatever tip you desire, and pipe evenly into the middle of each hot muffin. Let cool. Enjoy!

Nutrition Information

- Calories: 332.4
- Fiber: 4
- Cholesterol: 0
- Protein: 8.7
- Total Fat: 9.1
- Saturated Fat: 1.8
- Sodium: 326.7
- Sugar: 28.2
- Total Carbohydrate: 57.4

260. Oatmeal Zucchini Muffins

Serving: 12 muffins, 12 serving(s) | Prep: 10mins | Ready in:

Ingredients

- 1 cup oats
- 1 cup skim milk
- 1 cup flour
- 1/2 cup brown sugar
- 1/2 cup unsweetened applesauce
- 1 cup shredded zucchini
- 1 egg
- 1 teaspoon baking powder
- 1/2 teaspoon baking soda
- 1/2 teaspoon salt
- 1/2 teaspoon cinnamon

Direction

- Soak oats in milk for 1 hour.
- Add remaining ingredients, mix with fork until just moistened.
- Divide equally among 12 muffin tins that have been sprayed with non-stick spray or muffin liners.
- Bake in 400F for 25-30 minutes.

Nutrition Information

- Calories: 144
- Sodium: 202.8
- Total Carbohydrate: 28.3
- Cholesterol: 18
- Saturated Fat: 0.3
- Fiber: 1.9
- Sugar: 9.1
- Protein: 4.8
- Total Fat: 1.5

261. Oh So Yummy Peanut Butter Chocolate Chip Muffins

Serving: 12 large muffins, 12 serving(s) | Prep: 10mins | Ready in:

Ingredients

- 2 cups all-purpose flour
- 1 1/2 teaspoons baking soda
- 1/4 teaspoon salt
- 1/2 cup butter, softened
- 1 3/4 cups peanut butter, creamy
- 1 cup granulated sugar
- 2 large eggs
- 1/2 cup 1% low-fat milk
- 1/2 cup roasted peanuts, chopped
- 3/4 cup semi-sweet chocolate chips

Direction

- Preheat oven to 350°F Lightly grease 12 large muffin cups (16 medium size) or line with paper baking cups; set aside.
- In large bowl, combine flour, baking soda and salt and set aside.
- In another large mixing bowl, cream butter, peanut butter and sugar. Add eggs. Then gradually add milk and combine well.
- Add dry ingredients to peanut butter mixture and mix with a spoon until dry ingredients are moistened. Add chopped peanuts and chocolate chips and mix with a spoon. Mixture will be stiff. If you find it too stiff then add 1-2 tablespoons of milk to the batter. It is not to be runny though.
- Spoon batter into each muffin cup, filling cup. Bake 15-20 minutes or until lightly browned. Cool in muffin cups on wire rack for 5 minutes. Remove; cool completely.

Nutrition Information

- Calories: 551.4
- Saturated Fat: 11.7
- Sodium: 541
- Fiber: 4.2
- Total Carbohydrate: 49.2
- Cholesterol: 51.8
- Protein: 15.7
- Total Fat: 35.6
- Sugar: 26.8

262. Oil Free Bran Muffins

Serving: 12 muffins | Prep: 15mins | Ready in:

Ingredients

- 2 1/4 cups oat bran
- 1 tablespoon baking powder
- 1/4 cup brown sugar
- 1/2 cup seedless raisin
- 1 1/4 cups nonfat milk or 1 1/4 cups skim milk
- 2 egg whites
- 2 tablespoons light corn syrup
- 1 teaspoon ground cinnamon

Direction

- Preheat oven to 425°F.
- Mix the dry ingredients in a large bowl. Mix the milk, egg whites and corn syrup together and blend with the dry ingredients.
- Line muffin pans with paper baking cups and fill with batter divided equally. Bake 13 to 15 minutes. Test bran muffins doneness with toothpick.

Nutrition Information

- Calories: 102
- Sodium: 118.7
- Fiber: 3
- Total Carbohydrate: 25.4
- Cholesterol: 0.5
- Saturated Fat: 0.3
- Sugar: 10.6
- Protein: 4.7
- Total Fat: 1.3

263. Old Fashioned Baking Powder Biscuits

Serving: 8-10 biscuits, 8-10 serving(s) | Prep: 5mins | Ready in:

Ingredients

- 2 cups flour
- 2 teaspoons baking powder
- 1/2 teaspoon salt
- 1 cup cream
- 1 well-beaten egg

Direction

- Sift dry ingredients together; add cream and egg.
- Mix lightly together and roll out.
- Bake on a cookie sheet in a 400 degree oven about 20 minutes or until light brown.

Nutrition Information

- Calories: 210.8
- Saturated Fat: 6
- Sodium: 255.6
- Total Carbohydrate: 25.1
- Cholesterol: 59.6
- Protein: 4.7
- Total Fat: 10.2
- Fiber: 0.8
- Sugar: 0.2

264. One Banana Bread Muffins

Serving: 9-10 muffins | Prep: 10mins | Ready in:

Ingredients

- 1/4 cup butter
- 1 banana
- 1/4 cup sugar
- 1/3 cup brown sugar
- 1 tablespoon milk
- 1 egg
- 1/2 teaspoon vanilla
- 1/2 teaspoon baking soda
- 1/8 teaspoon salt
- 1 cup flour

Direction

- Preheat oven to 350°. Prep. Muffin tin, with butter/spray or liners.
- Melt Butter in Microwave for 30 seconds. Meanwhile, in a medium mixing bowl, mash your banana.
- Then in the same bowl add; sugar, brown sugar, milk, melted butter, egg. Then cream together.
- Once creamed, add Baking Soda, Salt, and flour. Mix well.
- Then fill the muffin tins 3/4 up, and place in the middle of the rack.
- Let them bake for 17 minutes, or until middle comes out clean with a knife.

Nutrition Information

- Calories: 169.6
- Protein: 2.4
- Sodium: 158.7
- Fiber: 0.7
- Saturated Fat: 3.5
- Sugar: 15.1
- Total Carbohydrate: 27.3
- Cholesterol: 34.5
- Total Fat: 5.9

265. Only Bran Muffins

Serving: 6 muffins | Prep: 10mins | Ready in:

Ingredients

- 1 cup oat bran
- 1 cup wheat bran
- 1 teaspoon baking soda or 1 teaspoon baking powder
- 1 cup nonfat plain yogurt
- 1 egg
- 1 egg white (optional)
- salt
- herbs

Direction

- Preheat oven to 375°F.
- Oil muffin pan. I usually spray each cup with a little bit of basil olive oil.
- Mix oat and wheat bran with baking soda/powder. Add salt or herbs to taste for savory muffins.
- In a separate bowl, mix yogurt and egg. Add an egg white for more moist muffins. Beat together well.
- Blend the yogurt mixture into bran mixture.
- Spoon into muffin pan.
- Bake for 10 to 20 minutes, depending on the size of each muffin. Overbaking can result in dry muffins (which aren't necessarily bad).
- Notes: I've added chopped onions and bell peppers, or baked them as a single loaf. Many variations have turned out well. Next time, I'll try a sweet version with orange peel and vanilla extract.

Nutrition Information

- Calories: 94.5
- Total Carbohydrate: 19.8
- Cholesterol: 36.1
- Saturated Fat: 0.6
- Sodium: 253.7
- Sugar: 3.5
- Protein: 7.6
- Total Fat: 2.4
- Fiber: 6.5

266. Oooey Gooey Incredibly Yummy Banana Cinnamon Toast

Serving: 2 serving(s) | Prep: 5mins | Ready in:

Ingredients

- 2 small bananas, peeled, halved and sliced
- 1/4 teaspoon ground cinnamon
- 2 fruit muffins or 2 fruit cake
- 2 almonds, blanched and chopped finely
- 1 tablespoon unsalted butter
- 2-3 tablespoons maple syrup or 2-3 tablespoons honey

Direction

- First, you got to slice the muffins into round slices and toast them lightly.
- Remove onto a plate Melt butter in a pan.
- Add banana slices and sauté till they brown a little and are soft.
- Stir in maple syrup, powdered cinnamon and the almonds.
- Mix lightly.
- Pour this mixture over the muffin slices.
- Remove onto a serving plate.
- Serve hot.
- Enjoy with full joy!

Nutrition Information

- Calories: 202.2
- Sugar: 24.3
- Protein: 1.5
- Total Fat: 6.9
- Saturated Fat: 3.8
- Cholesterol: 15.3
- Sodium: 8.5
- Fiber: 3
- Total Carbohydrate: 37

267. Orange Spiced Scones

Serving: 1 dozen | Prep: 15mins | Ready in:

Ingredients

- Scones
- 1 3/4 cups all-purpose flour
- 3 tablespoons sugar
- 2 1/2 teaspoons baking powder
- 2 teaspoons orange zest
- 1/3 cup cold butter
- 1/2 cup raisins
- 2 eggs, slightly beaten
- 4 -6 tablespoons half-and-half cream
- Orange Butter
- 1/2 cup butter, softened
- 2 tablespoons orange marmalade

Direction

- Heat oven to 400°F.
- Combine flour, sugar, baking powder and orange peel in medium bowl. Cut in 1/3 cup butter until mixture resembles fine crumbs. Stir in raisins, 1 beaten egg and just enough half half until mixture is moistened.
- Turn dough onto lightly floured surface; knead lightly 10 times. Roll into 9-inch circle; cut into 12 wedges. Place 1-inch apart onto ungreased baking sheet. Brush with remaining beaten egg. Bake for 10 to 12 minutes or until golden brown. Immediately remove from baking sheet.
- Stir together all orange butter ingredients in small bowl; serve with warm scones.

Nutrition Information

- Calories: 2848.2
- Total Fat: 172.7
- Sodium: 2196.3
- Sugar: 106.2
- Total Carbohydrate: 295.9
- Saturated Fat: 104.9
- Fiber: 9.3
- Cholesterol: 851.8
- Protein: 41

268. Peanut Butter Bran Muffins

Serving: 12 muffins | Prep: 10mins | Ready in:

Ingredients

- 50 g wheat bran
- 150 g flour
- 1 teaspoon salt
- 100 g brown sugar
- 1 tablespoon baking powder
- 150 g crunchy peanut butter
- 250 ml milk
- 2 eggs
- 50 g butter, melted
- 100 g semi-sweet chocolate chips

Direction

- Preheat oven to 400°F.
- In a large bowl, combine the bran, flour, salt, brown sugar, and baking powder.
- In a smaller bowl, cream peanut butter and milk. Stir in the eggs and the melted butter.
- Incorporate the peanut butter mix into the flour mixture. Add chocolate chips.
- Spoon into muffin pan and bake 15 to 20 minutes or until muffins are golden.

Nutrition Information

- Calories: 252.1
- Sugar: 13.7
- Cholesterol: 47
- Total Fat: 13.7
- Saturated Fat: 5.3
- Sodium: 392.9
- Fiber: 3.6
- Total Carbohydrate: 29.5
- Protein: 6.9

269. Peanut Butter Chocolate Chip Muffins

Serving: 12 serving(s) | Prep: 10mins | Ready in:

Ingredients

- 1 1/2 cups flour
- 1/3 cup sugar
- 2 1/2 teaspoons baking powder
- 1/2 cup peanut butter (chunky is recommended)
- 2 tablespoons margarine
- 2 eggs, beaten
- 3/4 cup low-fat milk
- 1/2 cup semi-sweet chocolate chips (I like the mini chips)

Direction

- Preheat oven to 400.
- Combine flour, sugar and baking powder. Cut peanut butter and margarine into dry mixture until coarse crumbs appear.
- In a small bowl combine eggs and milk. Add to flour mixture and stir until mixture is lumpy.
- Fold in chocolate chips.
- Spray muffin tins with cooking spray or use paper liners. Fill cups to 2/3 full.
- Bake 12-15 minutes until lightly browned.

Nutrition Information

- Calories: 211.1
- Total Fat: 10.5
- Sodium: 166.6
- Fiber: 1.5
- Saturated Fat: 3.1
- Sugar: 11.2
- Total Carbohydrate: 25.1
- Cholesterol: 36
- Protein: 6.2

270. Pearl's Granola Muffins

Serving: 12 serving(s) | Prep: 10mins | Ready in:

Ingredients

- 2 cups Bisquick
- 1 cup granola cereal
- 2 tablespoons honey
- 1 egg
- 2/3 cup milk
- 1/3 cup raisins

Direction

- Preheat oven to 400 degrees.
- Mix all ingredients together and beat for 1 minute.
- Line a muffin tin with paper liners and fill each liner about 2/3 full.
- Bake at 400 degrees for 15-18 minutes or until done in the middle.
- Serve warm.

Nutrition Information

- Calories: 172.9
- Saturated Fat: 1.7
- Sodium: 270.5
- Cholesterol: 19.9
- Protein: 4.2
- Total Fat: 6.5
- Fiber: 1.4
- Sugar: 9.7
- Total Carbohydrate: 24.8

271. Perfect Cornbread Muffins With Corn!

Serving: 48 mini muffins, 48 serving(s) | Prep: 5mins | Ready in:

Ingredients

- 1 1/4 cups flour
- 1 1/3 cups yellow cornmeal
- 1/3 cup sugar
- 1 1/2 teaspoons baking soda
- 1/2 teaspoon salt
- 4 tablespoons brown sugar
- 1 cup buttermilk (or 1 cup milk mixed with a few teaspoons lemon juice)
- 1/2 cup melted then cooled butter
- 1 egg, beaten
- 3/4-1 cup thawed frozen corn

Direction

- Grease mini muffin tins well then sprinkle the tins with a little flour to really get the tins stick proof! Preheat oven to 475°.
- Mix flour, corn meal, sugar, baking soda, salt and brown sugar together well.
- Mix milk, egg, and butter together in another bowl then stir in corn.
- Pour wet mixture into flour mixture and mix ONLY until just blended. Do not over mix!
- Scoop mixture into prepared tins and lower oven temp to 425 and bake for 8-12 minutes for mini muffin tins or about 15-20 for regular sized muffins OR until tooth pick comes out clean from the center muffin.
- Let cool on wire racks.

Nutrition Information

- Calories: 56.6
- Saturated Fat: 1.3
- Sodium: 88.9
- Sugar: 2.8
- Cholesterol: 9.2
- Fiber: 0.4
- Total Carbohydrate: 8.4
- Protein: 1
- Total Fat: 2.2

272. Pineapple Sweet Potato Muffins (Louisiana)

Serving: 16 serving(s) | Prep: 10mins | Ready in:

Ingredients

- 1 cup sweet potato, pureed
- 1 (8 ounce) can crushed pineapple, drained
- 1 teaspoon orange zest
- 2 eggs
- 2/3 cup granulated sugar
- 1/2 cup walnuts, chopped
- 2 cups all-purpose flour
- 1 tablespoon baking powder
- 1 teaspoon baking soda
- 1/2 teaspoon salt

Direction

- Preheat oven to 375 degrees F.
- In a medium bowl, combine sweet potatoes, pineapple, orange zest, eggs sugar, stirring until well combined, then stir in walnuts.
- In a large bowl, whisk together the flour, baking powder, baking soda salt, then pour wet ingredients into the dry ingredients fold until dry ingredients are JUST moistened.
- Spray muffin tins with nonstick cooking spray, then spoon 1/4 cup of the batter into each cup, if there isn't enough batter, put a small amount of water in the empty cups.
- Bake 16-20 minutes, then cool slightly serve.

Nutrition Information

- Calories: 138.2
- Total Fat: 3.1
- Saturated Fat: 0.5
- Sodium: 233.5
- Fiber: 1
- Total Carbohydrate: 24.9
- Cholesterol: 23.2
- Sugar: 10.9
- Protein: 3.1

273. Pistachio Orange Cherry Craisin Scones With Apricot Honey Butter

Serving: 8 Scones, 8 serving(s) | Prep: 15mins | Ready in:

Ingredients

- 2 cups all-purpose flour
- 1/3 cup sugar
- 2 1/2 teaspoons baking powder
- 1/3 cup of chopped pistachios
- 1/3 cup chopped cherry craisins
- 1 large orange, zest of
- 1/2 cup mandarin orange, drained
- 1/2 cup cold butter or 1/2 cup margarine
- 1/4 cup milk
- 1 slightly beaten egg
- 2 tablespoons sugar (for topping)
- apricot honey butter
- 1/2 cup butter (butter is fresher tasting) or 1/2 cup margarine (butter is fresher tasting)
- 1-2 tablespoon of raw wild natural honey
- 1/3 cup apricot preserves

Direction

- Preheat oven to 400 degrees. Mix flour, sugar, baking powder, pistachios, chopped cherry raisins, and orange zest together. Cut butter into small chunks and mix with dry ingredients. Use pastry cutter or fork and cut butter into dry ingredients until texture resembles coarse cornmeal. Mix milk, egg, and oranges together. Pour wet ingredients into dry ingredients. Stir until mixture pulls away from the sides. If mixture seems a little wet add a little more flour until it pulls away easily. Pour dough unto floured surface and knead 11 times. Remove dough carefully and place on cookie sheet forming a circle. Do not over handle the dough! Cut into 8 slices but don't separate pieces. Sprinkle with sugar and bake in oven until golden brown about 15-20 minutes. Serve warm with Apricot Honey Butter (recipe below).
- In small bowl whip butter until light and fluffy. Mix in honey and preserves by hand until blended. Adjust taste by adding a little more honey and preserves if necessary. Spread on warm scones. Store in air tight container in refrigerator.

Nutrition Information

- Calories: 467
- Sodium: 335.3
- Protein: 5.8
- Saturated Fat: 15.3
- Fiber: 1.9
- Sugar: 24.4
- Total Carbohydrate: 54
- Cholesterol: 85.3
- Total Fat: 26.6

274. Power Muffins

Serving: 12 serving(s) | Prep: 15mins | Ready in:

Ingredients

- 1 cup whole wheat flour
- 1 cup wheat bran
- 1/2 cup wheat germ
- 1 teaspoon baking powder
- 1 teaspoon baking soda
- 1/2 cup honey
- 1/4 cup applesauce
- 3/4 cup milk
- 1 egg, lightly beaten
- 1/4 cup walnuts
- 1/4 cup raisins
- 1/2 teaspoon nutmeg
- 1 teaspoon cinnamon

Direction

- Mix all the dry ingredients together, then add wet ingredients, stir well and put in greased muffin pans.
- SPRINKLE WITH CINNAMON AND BAKE AT 400 FOR FIFTEEN MINUTES.

Nutrition Information

- Calories: 150.6
- Saturated Fat: 0.8
- Sugar: 13.6
- Cholesterol: 19.8
- Total Fat: 3.5
- Sodium: 152.1
- Fiber: 4.4
- Total Carbohydrate: 29.3
- Protein: 4.8

275. Pumpkin Applesauce Muffins

Serving: 21 muffins, 21 serving(s) | Prep: 0S | Ready in:

Ingredients

- 1 1/2 tablespoons melted butter or 1 1/2 tablespoons cooking spray
- 3 1/3 cups all-purpose flour
- 2 teaspoons baking soda
- 1/2 teaspoon baking powder
- 2 teaspoons ground cinnamon
- 1/2 teaspoon ground cloves
- 1/2 teaspoon freshly grated nutmeg
- 1 teaspoon salt
- 8 tablespoons unsalted butter, softened
- 2 cups sugar
- 4 large eggs
- 1 cup applesauce
- 1 cup canned mashed pumpkin
- 1 teaspoon vanilla extract
- 2/3 cup apple juice or 2/3 cup cider or 2/3 cup orange juice
- 1 1/2 cups raisins

Direction

- Preheat oven to 375°F Grease 12 half-cup muffin cups with melted butter. In a medium bowl, combine flour, baking soda, baking powder, cinnamon, cloves, nutmeg, and salt; set aside.
- In a large mixing bowl, beat butter and sugar until creamy, 2 to 3 minutes. Beat in eggs, applesauce, pumpkin, and vanilla until blended. Add dry ingredients, alternating with the juice, beginning and ending with the dry mixture; mix until smooth. Fold in raisins.
- Spoon batter into prepared muffin cups, filling each cup two-thirds full. Bake on the center oven rack until a toothpick inserted in the center of each muffin comes out clean, 20 to 25 minutes. Remove from oven and allow muffins to cool in the pans several minutes; turn muffins out onto a rack. Serve muffins warm or at room temperature. Repeat steps 1 through 3 with remaining batter.

Nutrition Information

- Calories: 253
- Total Fat: 6.5
- Saturated Fat: 3.7
- Fiber: 1.2
- Sugar: 26.3
- Total Carbohydrate: 46.4
- Sodium: 264.4
- Cholesterol: 54.1
- Protein: 3.7

276. Pumpkin Bran Muffins

Serving: 12 muffins | Prep: 10mins | Ready in:

Ingredients

- 1 3/4 cups all-purpose flour
- 1/4 cup wheat germ
- 1/2 cup vegan sugar (or granulated sugar)

- 3 teaspoons baking powder
- 1/2 teaspoon salt
- 1/2 teaspoon cinnamon
- 1/4 teaspoon ground ginger
- 1/8 teaspoon ground cloves
- 1 teaspoon Ener-G Egg Substitute, mixed with 2 tablespoons water (or 2 egg whites or 1 whole egg)
- 1 cup pumpkin puree
- 1/2 cup raisins, chopped
- 1 cup shredded bran cereal
- 3/4 cup soymilk (or nonfat milk)
- 1/4 cup light corn syrup
- 1/4 cup sorghum molasses

Direction

- Preheat oven to 400 degrees.
- Spray cups of a 12-hole muffin tin with non-stick spray.
- Mix together in a large bowl dry ingredients.
- In a small bowl mix together wet ingredients.
- Blend two bowls together, mixing until ingredients are just moistened, about 20 stirs.
- Spoon batter, evenly divided, into muffin cups.
- Bake at 400 degrees for 20-25 minutes or until toothpick inserted comes out clean.
- Cool slightly in pan before transferring to wire rack to finish cooling (or serve warm as an option).

Nutrition Information

- Calories: 177.3
- Protein: 3.4
- Saturated Fat: 0.1
- Fiber: 1.4
- Sugar: 18
- Total Carbohydrate: 40.8
- Total Fat: 0.8
- Sodium: 204.6
- Cholesterol: 0

277. Pumpkin Granola Crumble Topped Muffins

Serving: 6-12 serving(s) | Prep: 6mins | Ready in:

Ingredients

- Topping
- 1/4 cup flour
- 1 1/2 tablespoons margarine
- 1 1/2 tablespoons sugar
- 1/4 teaspoon cinnamon
- Muffins
- 1 cup apple cinnamon granola cereal (I used Zoe's)
- 1/2 cup canned pumpkin, plus
- 2 tablespoons canned pumpkin
- 2 tablespoons apple butter
- 1/2 cup unsweetened applesauce
- 1/4 cup oil
- 1/2 teaspoon vanilla
- 3/4 cup whole wheat pastry flour
- 3/4 cup unbleached all-purpose flour
- 1/3 cup sugar
- 2 teaspoons baking powder
- 1/2 teaspoon baking soda
- 1/2 teaspoon salt
- 1/2 teaspoon cinnamon
- 2 tablespoons soymilk, or as needed

Direction

- Preheat oven to 400 degrees F.
- Spray either 6 large muffin baking cup pan or 12 small muffin cups with cooking spray.
- Make the topping, combine flour, cinnamon and sugar, cutting in margarine until mixture resembles coarse crumbs and set aside.
- In a large bowl, mix together the cereal, pumpkin puree, apple butter and applesauce.
- Set aside for 5 minutes, or until cereal is softened.
- Once cereal is soft, add the oil and vanilla.
- Stir together flours, sugar, baking powder, baking soda, salt and cinnamon in a medium bowl and set aside.

- Add the flour mixture to the pumpkin mixture, stirring until combined, you will need to add the soy milk to make it not such a stiff dough.
- Divide the mixture to muffin cups evenly.
- Sprinkle the muffins evenly with the topping.
- Bake for about 20 minutes, until golden and a toothpick inserted into the center of a muffin comes out clean.
- Place on cooling rack, cover with a tea towel for 5 minutes.
- After the five minutes, run a butter knife around the muffins, then remove very carefully, they are very soft and delicate.
- Cool completely, place in tupperware lined with a paper towel.
- Freeze after 1-2 days, wrapped in plastic wrap.

Nutrition Information

- Calories: 419.4
- Cholesterol: 0
- Total Fat: 17.6
- Fiber: 5.4
- Total Carbohydrate: 59.5
- Protein: 7.8
- Saturated Fat: 2.9
- Sodium: 524
- Sugar: 21.4

278. Pumpkin Oatmeal Muffins

Serving: 12 muffins, 6 serving(s) | Prep: 15mins | Ready in:

Ingredients

- 3/4 cup white flour
- 3/4 cup whole wheat flour
- 1 cup quick-cooking oats
- 3/4 cup brown sugar
- 1/2 cup raisins
- 1 tablespoon baking powder
- 1 teaspoon cinnamon
- 1/2 teaspoon nutmeg
- 1/4 teaspoon allspice
- 1 cup canned pumpkin
- 3/4 cup skim milk
- 1/3 cup canola oil
- 1 egg, lightly beaten

Direction

- Combine the dry ingredients in a large bowl (including raisins).
- Combine the wet ingredients in a separate bowl.
- Add the wet ingredients to the dry ingredients.
- Spray a muffin pan with non-stick spray and distribute batter evenly.
- Bake at 400 for about 20 minutes.

Nutrition Information

- Calories: 448.5
- Fiber: 5.5
- Sugar: 35.4
- Total Carbohydrate: 74.3
- Cholesterol: 35.9
- Saturated Fat: 1.5
- Sodium: 323.6
- Protein: 8.9
- Total Fat: 14.6

279. Pumpkin Whole Wheat Muffins

Serving: 12 muffins, 12 serving(s) | Prep: 10mins | Ready in:

Ingredients

- 1 cup all-purpose flour
- 3/4 cup whole wheat flour (soaked in 3/4 c of water)
- 1/3 cup sugar (or 1/2c if you prefer sweeter)

- 2 teaspoons baking powder
- 2 teaspoons pumpkin pie spice
- 1/2 teaspoon cinnamon
- 1/4 teaspoon ground ginger
- 1/4 teaspoon ground nutmeg
- 1/4 teaspoon baking soda
- 1/4 teaspoon salt
- 1 egg (beaten)
- 3/4 cup milk
- 2 tablespoons unsalted butter (melted)
- 3/4 cup pumpkin (canned)

Direction

- Preheat oven to 375 degrees.
- Butter and flour the sides of a muffin tin or, even easier, use muffin cups.
- In a small bowl blend together the wheat flour and 3/4 water. Set aside.
- In another bowl, combine the all-purpose flour with the remaining dry ingredients. Stir well.
- In a separate bowl combine the egg, melted butter, milk, and pumpkin. Mix well.
- Add the pumpkin mixture to the dry ingredients, then add the moistened wheat flour. Stir well until thoroughly combined. Fill each muffin cup about 2/3 full. Bake in oven for 15-20 minute.
- * Try topping with a mixture of brown sugar and cinnamon for a sweet crunch.

Nutrition Information

- Calories: 121.5
- Cholesterol: 24.9
- Protein: 3.2
- Saturated Fat: 1.8
- Fiber: 1.3
- Total Carbohydrate: 20.7
- Total Fat: 3.2
- Sodium: 149.6
- Sugar: 5.8

280. Pumpkin Oat Bran Muffins

Serving: 12 muffins | Prep: 0S | Ready in:

Ingredients

- 1 1/2 cups unprocessed oat bran
- 1/2 cup firmly packed brown sugar
- 1/2 cup all-purpose flour
- 2 teaspoons baking powder
- 1 teaspoon pumpkin pie spice
- 1/4 teaspoon salt
- 1 cup mashed pumpkin, , cooked
- 1/2 cup skim milk
- 2 egg whites, lightly beaten
- 2 tablespoons vegetable oil
- vegetable oil cooking spray

Direction

- Combine first six ingredients in a large bowl; stir well.
- Make a well in centre of mixture.
- Combine pumpkin and next three ingredients; stir well.
- Add to dry ingredients, stirring just until moistened.
- Spoon into muffin pans coated with cooking spray, filling ¾ full.
- Bake at 425 degrees for 20 minutes.
- Remove from pans immediately; serve warm or at room temperature.
- Banana Oat Bran Muffins: Substitute ¾ cup mashed ripe banana for pumpkin.
- Apple-Oat Bran Muffins: Substitute 1/2 cup minced apple for pumpkin.
- Substitute apple pie spice for pumpkin pie spice.
- Add 1 Tsp. ground cinnamon to dry ingredients.

Nutrition Information

- Calories: 113.2
- Fiber: 2

- Protein: 3.7
- Total Fat: 3.2
- Saturated Fat: 0.5
- Sodium: 127.5
- Sugar: 9.3
- Total Carbohydrate: 22.3
- Cholesterol: 0.2

281. Quick Easy Apple Muffins

Serving: 12 muffins | Prep: 10mins | Ready in:

Ingredients

- 1 egg
- 1 cup milk
- 1/4 cup rapeseed oil
- 2 apples
- 1 cup white flour
- 1 cup whole wheat flour
- 1/4 cup vanilla sugar
- 3 teaspoons baking powder
- 1 teaspoon cinnamon
- 1/8 teaspoon powdered ginger
- 1/2 teaspoon salt

Direction

- Preheat oven to 400°F/200°C Line muffin tin with muffin cups or grease the tin with some canola oil.
- Beat the egg in a mixing bowl.
- Add the milk and the rapeseed oil, stirring well.
- Peel the apples. I slice chunks around the core, but you can core them the traditional way. Chop the apples finely. Stir chopped apples into the mixture, blending thoroughly.
- Add the remaining ingredients. Stir until the dry ingredients are just moistened. (The batter will be very thick).
- Pour the batter into the cups. Bake for approximately 20-25 minutes.
- After baking, remove the muffins from the tin immediately. Serve hot and fresh.

Nutrition Information

- Calories: 107.8
- Total Fat: 1.6
- Sodium: 204.3
- Fiber: 2.2
- Saturated Fat: 0.7
- Sugar: 3.2
- Total Carbohydrate: 20.8
- Cholesterol: 18.4
- Protein: 3.7

282. Quick Applesauce Muffins

Serving: 12 serving(s) | Prep: 5mins | Ready in:

Ingredients

- 2 cups Bisquick
- 1/4 cup sugar
- 1 teaspoon cinnamon
- 1/2 cup applesauce
- 1/4 cup milk
- 1 egg
- 2 tablespoons sunflower oil
- TOPPING
- 1/4 cup sugar
- 1/4 teaspoon cinnamon
- 2 tablespoons butter or 2 tablespoons margarine, melted

Direction

- Preheat oven to 350°F.
- Combine Bisquick, 1/4 cup sugar, and 1 teaspoon cinnamon.
- Add applesauce, milk, egg and oil, and beat vigorously for 30 seconds.
- Fill greased muffin pans 2/3 full and bake 12-15 minutes.

- Cool slightly and remove from pans.
- Mix remaining sugar and cinnamon.
- Dip tops of muffins in melted butter, then in sugar-cinnamon mixture.

Nutrition Information

- Calories: 178.5
- Saturated Fat: 2.6
- Fiber: 0.7
- Total Carbohydrate: 24.4
- Cholesterol: 21.7
- Total Fat: 8.1
- Sodium: 244.3
- Sugar: 10.8
- Protein: 2.5

283. Quick Chive And Bacon Corn Muffins

Serving: 12 serving(s) | Prep: 12mins | Ready in:

Ingredients

- 14 ounces corn muffin mix
- 1 teaspoon chives, snipped
- 6 slices bacon, crisp-cooked, drained and crumbled
- 1/8 teaspoon black pepper

Direction

- Prepare muffin mix according to package directions.
- Fold in chives, bacon, and pepper.
- Pour into 12 greased muffin tins and bake at 400 degrees for 15 minutes or till done.
- Serve hot.

Nutrition Information

- Calories: 190.2
- Protein: 3.6
- Total Fat: 9.1
- Saturated Fat: 2.7
- Sodium: 461.9
- Fiber: 2.2
- Sugar: 6.7
- Total Carbohydrate: 23.1
- Cholesterol: 8.4

284. Quick Jalapeno Cheddar Muffins

Serving: 12 muffins, 4-6 serving(s) | Prep: 5mins | Ready in:

Ingredients

- 3 (8 1/2 ounce) boxes Jiffy corn muffin mix
- 3 eggs
- 1 cup cheddar cheese, grated
- 1/3 cup jalapeno pepper, chopped
- 1 cup cream or 1 cup half-and-half

Direction

- Combine all ingredients in a mixing bowl until a smooth batter is formed.
- Place 1/2 cup of batter in each well-greased muffin cup.
- Bake at 350 until golden brown, about 12-15 minutes.

Nutrition Information

- Calories: 1101.2
- Total Fat: 53.6
- Sugar: 37.5
- Total Carbohydrate: 128.5
- Protein: 25.8
- Saturated Fat: 24.3
- Sodium: 2256.2
- Fiber: 12
- Cholesterol: 258.2

285. Quick Mini Monkey Breads

Serving: 12 muffins, 12 serving(s) | Prep: 10mins | Ready in:

Ingredients

- 3/4 cup granulated sugar
- 2 teaspoons ground cinnamon
- 2 (7 1/2 ounce) cans refrigerated buttermilk biscuits
- 1/2 cup butter or 1/2 cup margarine, melted
- 3/4 cup brown sugar, packed

Direction

- Pre-heat oven to 400 degrees. Grease or spray muffin tins.
- Mix granulated sugar and cinnamon in 1-gallon bag. Cut each biscuit into quarters (kitchen shears or a pizza cutter make this a cinch!); Shake quarters in bag to coat.
- Using a 12 cup muffin tin, place 6-7 pieces of the coated biscuit dough into each muffin cup.
- Mix brown sugar and melted butter and pour over biscuit pieces.
- Bake at 400 degrees for 12-14 minutes until golden brown. Invert mini monkey breads onto a plate and serve warm.

Nutrition Information

- Calories: 283.8
- Sodium: 426.2
- Cholesterol: 20.7
- Total Fat: 12.5
- Saturated Fat: 6.1
- Fiber: 0.5
- Sugar: 28.5
- Total Carbohydrate: 41.7
- Protein: 2.5

286. Quick Vegan Pumpkin Spice Scones With Flax Seeds

Serving: 10 scones, 10 serving(s) | Prep: 10mins | Ready in:

Ingredients

- 3 cups all-purpose flour
- 2 tablespoons baking powder
- 1/4 cup sugar
- 1/2 teaspoon salt
- 1/2 teaspoon pumpkin pie spice
- 1/3 cup sunflower oil
- 1 1/2 cups pumpkin puree
- 1 teaspoon apple cider vinegar
- 2 teaspoons brown flax seeds

Direction

- Sift all the dry ingredients in a large bowl together.
- Mix the wet ingredients with the flax seeds in another bowl, then add to the large bowl with the dry ingredients.
- Mix the dough by hand, but don't over-mix. It should be a little floury and crumbly.
- Grease a cookie sheet with cooking spray then form small discs with the dough, about 9-10 of them, and space them out evenly.
- Bake at 400F for 12-15 minutes or until set.

Nutrition Information

- Calories: 230
- Total Fat: 7.9
- Saturated Fat: 1
- Sodium: 335.3
- Sugar: 5.3
- Total Carbohydrate: 35.7
- Cholesterol: 0
- Fiber: 1.3
- Protein: 4.2

287. Quick Whipping Cream Biscuits

Serving: 2 dozen | Prep: 10mins | Ready in:

Ingredients

- 1 cup butter
- 4 cups self-rising flour
- 1 3/4-2 cups whipping cream
- 1/2 cup butter, melted

Direction

- Cut 1 cup butter into flour with a pastry blender or fork until crumbly. Add whipping cream, stirring just until dry ingredients are moistened.
- Turn dough out onto a light floured surface and knead lightly 3 or 4 times. Roll or pat dough to 3/4 inch thickness.
- Cut with a 2-inch round cutter, and place biscuits on a lightly greased baking sheet.
- Bake at 400 degrees F. for 13-15 minutes. Brush warm biscuits with 1/2 cup melted butter.

Nutrition Information

- Calories: 2824.2
- Saturated Fat: 135.8
- Sugar: 0.9
- Total Carbohydrate: 191.5
- Cholesterol: 651.3
- Total Fat: 217.6
- Protein: 30.4
- Sodium: 4469.7
- Fiber: 6.8

288. Quick Yogurt Scones

Serving: 12 serving(s) | Prep: 15mins | Ready in:

Ingredients

- 3 cups all-purpose flour
- 2 teaspoons baking powder
- 2 teaspoons baking soda
- 1/2 teaspoon salt
- 6 tablespoons cold margarine
- 2 tablespoons brown sugar
- 1 1/4 cups plain low-fat yogurt
- 2 eggs
- 1/2 cup raisins

Direction

- Preheat oven to 400 degrees. Grease a large baking sheet.
- Sift together the flour, baking powder, baking soda, and salt. With a pastry cutter, cut the flour mixture together with the cold margarine and brown sugar until well blended.
- In a small bowl beat together the yogurt and 1 egg. Pour into the pastry mixture. Add raisins and stir just until mixed.
- Drop by rounded 1/4-cup measures onto the prepared baking sheet. Beat remaining egg and brush onto tops of scones. Bake for 12-15 minutes. Serve warm.

Nutrition Information

- Calories: 219.6
- Fiber: 1.1
- Sugar: 7.7
- Cholesterol: 32.5
- Protein: 5.9
- Total Fat: 7.2
- Saturated Fat: 1.8
- Sodium: 465.3
- Total Carbohydrate: 33

289. Quick Zucchini Carrot Muffins

Serving: 16 muffins | Prep: 5mins | Ready in:

Ingredients

- 1 (18 1/2 ounce) package carrot cake mix
- 1 egg
- 1/2 cup applesauce
- 1/4 cup vegetable oil
- 1 1/2 cups zucchini, shredded
- 1/2 cup raisins
- 1/2 cup pecans, chopped

Direction

- In a large mixing bowl, combine the cake mix, egg, applesauce and oil.
- Mix well, stir in zucchini, raisins and pecans.
- Fill greased or paper-lined muffin cups 3/4 full.
- Bake at 350 degrees for 25-30 minutes.

Nutrition Information

- Calories: 215.7
- Total Fat: 9.4
- Total Carbohydrate: 32
- Cholesterol: 13.2
- Protein: 2.7
- Saturated Fat: 1.2
- Sodium: 194.1
- Fiber: 0.7
- Sugar: 3

290. Really Good Low Cal, Low Fat, Healthy Blueberry Oatmeal Muffins

Serving: 12 serving(s) | Prep: 10mins | Ready in:

Ingredients

- 1 cup whole wheat flour
- 1/3 cup splenda brown sugar substitute
- 3 teaspoons baking powder
- 1/4 teaspoon cinnamon
- 1 cup oats
- 1/2 cup egg white
- 1/3 cup canola oil
- 1/3 cup 2% low-fat milk
- 1 teaspoon vanilla
- 1 cup blueberries (fresh or frozen)

Direction

- Preheat oven 400.
- Combine fist five ingredients in bowl and whisk until mixed well.
- Stir in all remaining ingredients except blueberries and mix.
- Gently fold in blueberries and fill lined muffin cups to 3/4 full.
- Bake for 18 - 20 minutes.

Nutrition Information

- Calories: 130.6
- Protein: 3.9
- Total Fat: 6.8
- Sodium: 111.3
- Sugar: 1.8
- Saturated Fat: 0.6
- Fiber: 2.2
- Total Carbohydrate: 14.3
- Cholesterol: 0.5

291. Rice Krispies Muffins

Serving: 24 muffins, 12 serving(s) | Prep: 10mins | Ready in:

Ingredients

- 1/4 cup butter
- 1 cup dark chocolate
- 1/4 cup syrup
- 5 cups Rice Krispies

Direction

- Melt butter, chocolate and sirop.
- Pour over the rice krispies and blend carefully.
- Put into muffin paper cups and cool for at least 4 hours.

Nutrition Information

- Calories: 149.5
- Fiber: 1.9
- Cholesterol: 10.2
- Sodium: 107.2
- Sugar: 2.6
- Total Carbohydrate: 17.2
- Protein: 2.3
- Total Fat: 9.7
- Saturated Fat: 6

292. Rosemary Garlic Buttery Biscuits

Serving: 12 drop biscuits | Prep: 10mins | Ready in:

Ingredients

- 1 cup flour
- 2 garlic cloves, crushed and minced
- 1 teaspoon rosemary, crushed and minced
- 1/4 teaspoon kosher salt
- 2 teaspoons baking powder
- 1/4 teaspoon cream of tartar
- 3 teaspoons sugar
- 1/8 teaspoon garlic powder
- 1/4 cup butter, chilled
- 1/2 cup milk
- 1/8 cup sharp cheddar cheese, shredded
- 1/8 cup monterey jack cheese, shredded
- 2 tablespoons butter, melted
- 1/4 teaspoon garlic powder
- 1/2 teaspoon rosemary, crushed and minced

Direction

- Combine flour, salt, baking powder, cream of tartar, sugar and 1/8 teaspoons garlic powder in a mixing bowl.
- Cut in butter using a pastry blender.
- Mix milk, cheeses, rosemary and garlic into dough.
- Drop by large spoonfuls onto greased baking sheet.
- Bake at 425°F for 10-12 minutes.
- Mix melted butter 1/4 teaspoons garlic powder, and 1/2 teaspoon rosemary together and brush on warm biscuits as soon as you remove them from the oven.

Nutrition Information

- Calories: 110.2
- Saturated Fat: 4.4
- Sugar: 1.1
- Total Carbohydrate: 10
- Cholesterol: 19
- Protein: 2.1
- Total Fat: 7
- Sodium: 156.7
- Fiber: 0.3

293. Rumford's Baking Powder Biscuits

Serving: 8-10 biscuits | Prep: 10mins | Ready in:

Ingredients

- 2 cups sifted unbleached white flour
- 3 teaspoons aluminum-free baking powder
- 1 teaspoon salt
- 6 tablespoons shortening (lard or refined coconut oil can be substituted)
- 2/3 cup milk (I tried buttermilk and used closer to 3/4 cup)

Direction

- Note: I used a KitchenAid stand up mixer to prep the dough.
- PREHEAT oven to 450 degrees.
- Sift flour, baking powder and salt together in a large bowl.
- Cut in shortening until mixture resemble coarse meal.

- Add milk to make a soft dough.
- Turn dough out on a floured surface and knead *gently* for 30 seconds.
- Roll out to 1/2 inch to 3/4 inch thickness.
- Use a cookie cutter to cut out into rounds. I used a 3-inch diameter Fiestaware tumbler cup, top floured.
- Place on greased or parchment-lined baking sheet.
- Bake approximately 12-15 minutes or until light golden.

Nutrition Information

- Calories: 212.5
- Total Carbohydrate: 25.2
- Cholesterol: 2.9
- Saturated Fat: 2.9
- Sugar: 0.1
- Sodium: 437.4
- Fiber: 0.8
- Protein: 3.9
- Total Fat: 10.7

294. Salba Banana Coconut Muffins

Serving: 6 muffins, 6 serving(s) | Prep: 5mins | Ready in:

Ingredients

- 2 tablespoons coconut oil
- 3 eggs, room temperature
- 1/4 cup mashed banana (1 small ripe banana)
- 1 teaspoon vanilla extract
- 1/4 teaspoon salt
- 1/4 cup coconut flour
- 2 tablespoons salba seeds
- 1 tablespoon shredded coconut (I use unsweetened)
- 1/2 teaspoon cinnamon
- 1/4 teaspoon baking powder
- 2 tablespoons raisins (optional)

Direction

- Preheat oven to 400°F Spray muffin tins with cooking spray.
- Mix together oil, eggs, banana, vanilla and salt.
- Add coconut flour, Salba seeds, shredded coconut, cinnamon and baking powder and whisk together until smooth.
- Fold in raisins, if using-I did not.
- Pour into muffin cups. Bake 15 minutes or until toothpick inserted in the center of muffins comes out clean. I had to bake about 5 minutes longer.

Nutrition Information

- Calories: 91.5
- Sodium: 149.7
- Sugar: 1.8
- Cholesterol: 105.8
- Protein: 3.3
- Total Fat: 7.4
- Saturated Fat: 5
- Fiber: 0.4
- Total Carbohydrate: 3.1

295. Salmon Orzo Salad And Cheesy Herb Muffins

Serving: 8 serving(s) | Prep: 20mins | Ready in:

Ingredients

- Salmon Orzo Salad
- 1/2 cup three cheese Italian salad dressing
- 1/2 cup plain yogurt
- 1/4 cup mayonnaise
- 2 tablespoons milk
- 1/4 cup grated parmesan cheese
- 1 (16 ounce) package orzo pasta
- 1 -2 cooked salmon fillets or 1 -2 steak
- 2 cups grape tomatoes
- 1 yellow bell pepper, chopped

- 1 green bell pepper, chopped
- 1 cup diced havarti cheese or 1 cup muenster cheese
- 1 cup frozen baby peas
- Cheesy Herbed Muffins
- 1/4 cup minced onion
- 1/4 cup minced parsley
- 2 teaspoons dill seeds
- 1 tablespoon minced fresh thyme
- 2 teaspoons minced garlic cloves
- 1/2 cup flour
- 1/2 cup whole wheat flour
- 2 tablespoons sugar
- 2 teaspoons baking powder
- 1 teaspoon baking soda
- 1/4 teaspoon salt
- 1/2 teaspoon dill weed
- 1/8 teaspoon white pepper
- 1/3 cup butter
- 1 cup diced havarti cheese
- 1/4 cup grated parmesan cheese
- 1 egg
- 1 cup buttermilk

Direction

- SALMON ORZO SALAD:
- Bring a large pot of water to a boil. In large bowl, combine salad dressing, yogurt, mayonnaise, milk, and Parmesan cheese and mix well.
- Flake salmon and add to dressing mixture along with tomatoes, bell peppers, and cheese and stir gently. Top with peas; do not stir.
- Cook pasta according to package directions until al dente. Drain and add to salad in bowl; stir gently to combine. Cover and chill for 2-3 hours to blend flavors before serving.
- CHEESY HERBED MUFFINS:
- Preheat oven to 400°F. Grease 12 muffin cups with unsalted butter and set aside. Combine onion, parsley, dill seed, thyme, and garlic in small bowls; set aside.
- In large bowl, combine flour, whole wheat flour, sugar, baking powder, baking soda, salt, and dill weed and mix until blended; there will be a few lumps. Fill prepared muffin cups 3/4 full. Sprinkle each muffin with the onion mixture and lightly press into batter.
- Bake muffins at 400°F for 17-22 minutes or until muffins are firm and light golden brown. Cool 1 minute in pan, then remove from pans and cool for 30 minutes on wire racks; serve warm. 12 muffins.
- To reheat in the microwave, place muffins on a microwave-safe plate and cover with microwave-safe paper towel. Microwave on HIGH for 10-15 seconds per muffins; let stand 1 minute, then serve.

Nutrition Information

- Calories: 564.1
- Saturated Fat: 8.3
- Fiber: 5
- Sugar: 11.3
- Total Carbohydrate: 70.7
- Total Fat: 20.8
- Protein: 24.4
- Sodium: 774.2
- Cholesterol: 73

296. Sausage Cheese English Muffins

Serving: 18 serving(s) | Prep: 15mins | Ready in:

Ingredients

- 2 lbs bulk sausage, good quality (I use Jimmy Dean)
- 3 (5 ounce) jarsKraft old English cheese
- 18 English muffins

Direction

- Brown sausage in large skillet or saucepan and drain.
- Combine sausage and cheese and stir until cheese is completely melted.
- Split English muffins.

- Divide mixture equally by placing even amounts onto bottoms of English muffins.
- Replace tops and wrap with plastic wrap.
- Store in freezer bag and freeze until needed.
- To use: Microwave for 1 minute.

Nutrition Information

- Calories: 245.9
- Protein: 12.6
- Total Fat: 10.3
- Sodium: 498
- Fiber: 2
- Total Carbohydrate: 25.2
- Saturated Fat: 2.9
- Sugar: 2
- Cholesterol: 36.8

297. Sausage, Egg Cheese Biscuits

Serving: 2 biscuits, 6 serving(s) | Prep: 5mins | Ready in:

Ingredients

- 2 cups Bisquick
- 1 lb cooked crumbled sausage
- 1 egg
- 2/3 cup plain yogurt
- 2/3 cup shredded cheese
- 1/2 teaspoon salt

Direction

- Combine all ingredients well in a large mixing bowl.
- Form patties about 1/2" thick and 3" diameter.
- Place patties on a greased cookie sheet about 1" apart.
- Bake at 450 for 11 - 15 minutes, or until golden brown.
- Enjoy!
- Substitutions: sausage: you could use vegetarian sausage without browning.
- Yogurt: milk or sour cream or buttermilk.

Nutrition Information

- Calories: 494.9
- Total Carbohydrate: 31.2
- Protein: 16.9
- Total Fat: 33.1
- Fiber: 0.9
- Sugar: 6.3
- Saturated Fat: 11.8
- Sodium: 1460.6
- Cholesterol: 87.3

298. Savory Breakfast Muffins.

Serving: 12 serving(s) | Prep: 10mins | Ready in:

Ingredients

- 2 cups whole wheat flour
- 1 cup all-purpose flour
- 1 tablespoon baking powder
- 1/2 teaspoon baking soda
- 1/2 teaspoon fresh ground pepper
- 1/4 teaspoon salt
- 2 eggs
- 1 1/3 cups buttermilk
- 3 tablespoons extra-virgin olive oil
- 2 tablespoons butter, melted
- 1 cup scallion, thinly sliced (about 1 bunch)
- 3/4 cup Canadian bacon, diced (3 ounces)
- 1/2 cup cheddar cheese, grated
- 1/2 cup red bell pepper, finely diced

Direction

- Preheat oven to 400°F Coat 12 muffin cups with cooking spray.
- Combine whole-wheat flour, all-purpose flour, baking powder, baking soda, pepper and salt in a large bowl.
- Whisk eggs, buttermilk, oil and butter in a medium bowl. Fold in scallions, bacon, cheese

and bell pepper. Make a well in the center of the dry ingredients. Add the wet ingredients and mix with a rubber spatula until just moistened. Scoop the batter into the prepared pan (the cups will be very full).
- Bake the muffins until the tops are golden brown, 20 to 22 minutes. Let cool in the pan for 5 minutes. Loosen the edges and turn the muffins out onto a wire rack to cool slightly before serving.
- Reheat Run Bake muffins on weekends and enjoy the leftovers for grab-and-go weekday breakfasts. Wrap leftover muffins individually in plastic wrap, place in a plastic storage container or ziplock bag and freeze for up to 1 month. To thaw, remove plastic wrap, wrap in a paper towel and microwave on High for 30 to 60 seconds.

Nutrition Information

- Calories: 199.9
- Protein: 7.1
- Cholesterol: 42.1
- Saturated Fat: 3.2
- Sodium: 280.5
- Fiber: 2.8
- Sugar: 1.9
- Total Carbohydrate: 25.1
- Total Fat: 8.5

299. Savory Cheese, Cranberry And Herb Mini Muffins

Serving: 36 min-muffins, 12 serving(s) | Prep: 10mins | Ready in:

Ingredients

- 1/4 cup canola oil
- 1/2 cup chopped scallion
- 1/4 teaspoon dried thyme
- 1/4 teaspoon dried oregano
- 1/4 teaspoon dried sage
- 1 cup all-purpose white flour
- 1 cup whole wheat pastry flour
- 1 tablespoon baking powder
- 1 teaspoon salt
- 1 pinch cayenne
- 1/2 cup dried cranberries
- 1 cup grated sharp cheddar cheese
- 1 egg
- 1 cup low-fat milk

Direction

- Preheat oven to 400°F.
- In a skillet, heat oil over medium heat. Add scallions, thyme, oregano and sage. Cook for 2 minutes until fragrant. Remove from heat and set aside.
- Combine both flours with baking powder, salt and cayenne. Stir in the cranberries and cheese.
- In a large mixing bowl, beat egg lightly. Whisk in the milk.
- Whisk the cooked scallions and herbs, including all the oil, into the milk and egg.
- Fold the dry ingredients into the egg and milk, mixing until just combined.
- Scoop batter into lightly greased mini-muffin tins.
- Bake for 15 to 18 minutes or until lightly browned and a toothpick inserted in the middle comes out clean.
- Remove from the oven and let cool for a few minutes before taking muffins out of the tin. Serve warm.

Nutrition Information

- Calories: 168.6
- Saturated Fat: 2.6
- Fiber: 1.8
- Sugar: 1.5
- Total Carbohydrate: 17.5
- Cholesterol: 28.5
- Total Fat: 8.6
- Sodium: 359.3
- Protein: 6.1

300. Savory Herb Biscuits (Sage And Caraway) With Garlic Butter

Serving: 16 1 3/4, 16 serving(s) | Prep: 10mins | Ready in:

Ingredients

- biscuits
- 2 tablespoons extra virgin olive oil
- 2 cups flour
- 1 1/4 teaspoons caraway seeds
- 1/2 teaspoon sage leaf, crumbled
- 1/4 teaspoon dry mustard
- 3 teaspoons baking powder
- 1 teaspoon salt
- 1/4 cup shortening
- 3/4 cup 2% low-fat milk
- garlic butter
- 1/4 cup butter, melted
- 1/4 teaspoon garlic powder

Direction

- Preheat oven to 450°F.
- Lightly grease a cookie sheet with olive oil.
- In a large mixing bowl, combine flour, caraway seed, sage, mustard, baking powder, and salt; mix well with a fork.
- Cut in shortening using a pastry blender or a fork until dough resembles coarse meal.
- Gently stir in most of the milk until well blended (if dough is not soft easy to roll, add just enough milk to make it pliable; too much milk will make dough sticky, but the biscuits will be dry if you don't add enough).
- Gather dough into a ball, and knead gently for about 30 seconds on a lightly floured surface.
- Roll out dough into a circle about 1/2" thick.
- Cut using a floured 1 1/2" biscuit cutter or cookie cutter.
- Gather up scraps of dough and re-roll and cut out remaining biscuits.
- Place on greased cookie sheet about 1/2 inch apart.
- Bake for 10-12 minutes (until golden brown).
- Mix garlic powder in butter.
- Serve biscuits hot with garlic butter.

Nutrition Information

- Calories: 132.6
- Sodium: 238.9
- Sugar: 0.6
- Total Carbohydrate: 12.8
- Saturated Fat: 3
- Fiber: 0.5
- Cholesterol: 8.5
- Protein: 2.1
- Total Fat: 8.2

301. Scone Recipe (C.w.a.)

Serving: 36 scones | Prep: 10mins | Ready in:

Ingredients

- 750 g self raising flour (6 cups)
- 1 teaspoon salt
- 250 ml cream (1 cup)
- 500 ml milk (approx)

Direction

- Sift flour and salt really well together.
- Add sufficient enough milk and cream gradually, to make a firm but not dry mixture (just enough milk to make a dough, which is easy to handle and not too sticky, without too much extra flour on the board).
- Roll the mixture one way lightly. Cut and place scone shapes on a cold tray and brush tops with a little milk or melted butter.
- Bake in an oven set at 220C for 8 to 10 minutes.

Nutrition Information

- Calories: 124.2
- Sugar: 0.1
- Total Fat: 2.9
- Saturated Fat: 1.7
- Sodium: 74.2
- Fiber: 0.7
- Total Carbohydrate: 20.7
- Cholesterol: 9.8
- Protein: 3.3

302. Scotch Pancakes Or Drop Scones

Serving: 18 pancakes | Prep: 20mins | Ready in:

Ingredients

- 120 g self raising flour
- 30 g caster sugar
- 1 pinch salt
- 1 egg
- 1/4 pint milk

Direction

- Mix or sift the flour, sugar and salt together.
- Make a well/hollow in the flour, then add the egg and milk into it.
- Mix, incorporating the flour from around the well until you have a thick, smooth batter that drops from the spoon like thick cream. (If you want to add any extras, do it now.).
- Heat a frying pan with a little butter or oil, wipe off if there's too much.
- Drop teaspoonfuls of batter into the pan. Leave enough room between them to maneuver a fish slice/your preferred pancake turning implement.
- When bubbles appear, turn the pancakes over and cook until lightly browned and no longer battery.
- Serve with butter, jam or honey or anything you fancy.

Nutrition Information

- Calories: 45.2
- Sodium: 16
- Fiber: 0.2
- Sugar: 1.7
- Total Carbohydrate: 8.4
- Cholesterol: 12.7
- Total Fat: 0.6
- Saturated Fat: 0.2
- Protein: 1.4

303. Season's Severed Finger Banana Muffins (Low Fat)

Serving: 12 muffins | Prep: 10mins | Ready in:

Ingredients

- 2 cups whole wheat flour
- 1/2 cup sugar or 1/2 cup brown sugar
- 1 teaspoon baking powder
- 1 teaspoon baking soda
- 1 dash salt
- 1 egg
- 3 bananas
- 1 cup applesauce (chunky)
- 1/8 cup oil
- 1 teaspoon orange juice concentrate
- 1 cup nuts, chopped (optional)
- sugar (optional)
- cinnamon (optional)
- strawberry jam (optional)

Direction

- Use either candy applesauce which is already red or add enough red food coloring to achieve a "red" color.
- Stir together all the dry ingredients and then mix in the wet ingredients - making sure not to over mix.

- Spoon into a lightly greased muffin tin. You can also at this stage sprinkle with cinnamon and sugar or lightly spoon strawberry jam on top.
- Bake at 350 degrees for 20-25 minutes.

Nutrition Information

- Calories: 169.6
- Fiber: 3.5
- Sugar: 12.2
- Total Carbohydrate: 34.1
- Protein: 3.6
- Total Fat: 3.2
- Saturated Fat: 0.6
- Sodium: 161.2
- Cholesterol: 17.6

304. Self Rising Biscuits

Serving: 12 biscuits, 12 serving(s) | Prep: 15mins | Ready in:

Ingredients

- 2 cups self rising flour
- 2/3 cup milk
- 1 large egg
- 3 tablespoons melted shortening

Direction

- Mix together.
- Place onto floured surface.
- Roll to 1/2 inch thickness.
- Cut.
- Bake at 450 for 10 to 12 minutes.

Nutrition Information

- Calories: 116.9
- Saturated Fat: 1.3
- Sodium: 277.1
- Fiber: 0.6
- Cholesterol: 19.5
- Protein: 3
- Total Fat: 4.3
- Sugar: 0.1
- Total Carbohydrate: 16.1

305. Seriously Strong Scottish Cheese Scones

Serving: 4 serving(s) | Prep: 10mins | Ready in:

Ingredients

- 1 1/2 cups self raising flour
- 1 ounce salted butter
- 1 large egg
- 2 tablespoons whole milk
- 4 ounces mull of kintyre cheese or 4 ounces scottish seriously strong cheddar cheese
- 1/3 teaspoon salt
- 1 1/4 teaspoons mustard powder
- 1 pinch cayenne pepper

Direction

- Mix the flour, salt and pepper together.
- Massage in the butter and then slowly mix in the grated cheese.
- Beat the egg and add in the milk; add mixture to the dry ingredients to create a soft, elastic dough.
- Roll out the mixture on a lightly floured surface. Cut into round shapes and place on a well-greased tray.
- Brush the top with milk and sprinkle a little extra cheese and pepper on top.
- Bake in a pre-heated oven in the center at 400 until golden brown.

Nutrition Information

- Calories: 249.2
- Sugar: 0.7
- Cholesterol: 68.9

- Total Fat: 8
- Saturated Fat: 4.3
- Sodium: 255.9
- Fiber: 1.4
- Total Carbohydrate: 36.6
- Protein: 7

306. Simple And Scrumptious Banana Bread

Serving: 2 loaves or about 18 muffins, 18 serving(s) | Prep: 5mins | Ready in:

Ingredients

- 4 eggs
- 1/4 cup applesauce (veggie or coconut oil can be substituted)
- 1/4 cup coconut oil (veggie oil can be substituted)
- 1/2 cup white sugar
- 1/2 cup brown sugar (white sugar can be substituted)
- 4 -6 overripe bananas, mashed (as in BLACK they're so ripe)
- 2 teaspoons vanilla
- 2 cups white whole wheat flour (all-purpose works as well)
- 2 teaspoons baking soda
- 1 teaspoon salt

Direction

- 1. Mash bananas.
- 2. Mix sugar and all wet ingredients in to the bananas; coconut oil may need to be heated slightly to get it to liquid state before mixing.
- 3. Mix the flour, soda, and salt in with the wet mixture, just until combined.
- 4. Pour into greased loaf or cupcake pans (or use liners) and bake at 350 degrees for one hour (loaves) or 25 minutes (cupcakes). Check for doneness and adjust cooking times as necessary; everyone's oven is a bit different.

- This bread is even better with any of these added: a bit of cinnamon, semisweet chocolate chips, pecans or walnuts, or cream cheese frosting.

Nutrition Information

- Calories: 159.4
- Sugar: 14.8
- Protein: 3.5
- Total Fat: 4.5
- Fiber: 2.1
- Total Carbohydrate: 28
- Cholesterol: 41.3
- Saturated Fat: 3
- Sodium: 288.1

307. Simple, Healthy Pumpkin Muffins

Serving: 24 muffins | Prep: 5mins | Ready in:

Ingredients

- 2/3 cup canned pumpkin
- 1 egg white
- 2/3 cup water
- 1 spice cake mix

Direction

- Preheat oven to 350 and line a muffin pan with cupcake papers.
- Mix all ingredients and spoon into papers 3/4 full.
- Bake 12-18 min or until a toothpick comes out clean.

Nutrition Information

- Calories: 77.9
- Saturated Fat: 0.6
- Sodium: 131.4
- Sugar: 8.2

- Total Carbohydrate: 13.3
- Total Fat: 2.4
- Fiber: 0.5
- Cholesterol: 0
- Protein: 1

308. Simple, Low Fat Banana Muffins

Serving: 12 12 muffins, 8-10 serving(s) | Prep: 10mins | Ready in:

Ingredients

- 1 1/2 cups whole wheat pastry flour
- 1 teaspoon baking soda
- 1 teaspoon baking powder
- 1/2 teaspoon salt
- 3 large bananas, mashed
- 1 large egg
- 3/4 cup brown sugar
- 1/3 cup unsweetened applesauce
- 1 1/2 teaspoons almond extract

Direction

- Preheat oven to 350 degrees and spray muffin tins with nonstick spray.
- Place all dry ingredients in a bowl and mix. Combine remaining ingredients and add to dry mixture folding together with a spatula until just combined. Watch the muffins carefully and remove from oven when still slightly moist in the middle.

Nutrition Information

- Calories: 216
- Protein: 4.4
- Total Carbohydrate: 49.5
- Fiber: 3.9
- Sugar: 27.4
- Cholesterol: 23.2
- Total Fat: 1.3

- Saturated Fat: 0.3
- Sodium: 363.9

309. Six Week Muffins

Serving: 6 dozen | Prep: 15mins | Ready in:

Ingredients

- 1 (15 ounce) box Raisin Bran cereal
- 3 cups sugar
- 5 cups flour
- 5 teaspoons baking soda
- 2 teaspoons cinnamon
- 2 teaspoons salt
- 4 beaten eggs
- 1 cup melted margarine
- 1 quart buttermilk

Direction

- Mix raisin bran, sugar, flour, soda, cinnamon and salt in large bowl.
- Stir in beaten eggs, margarine, and buttermilk.
- Mix well.
- Store, covered, in refrigerator.
- To use, bake at 400 for 15-20 minutes.
- Will keep in fridge for 6 weeks.
- Sugarless version: I think you could take off half the sugar, add the sugar replacement, and 1 t baking soda.

Nutrition Information

- Calories: 1378.9
- Sodium: 2819.3
- Total Carbohydrate: 242.6
- Protein: 26.8
- Saturated Fat: 7.8
- Fiber: 11.7
- Sugar: 131
- Cholesterol: 147.5
- Total Fat: 37.8

310. Skillet Cornbread

Serving: 4-6 serving(s) | Prep: 15mins | Ready in:

Ingredients

- 1 1/2 cups white cornmeal
- 3 tablespoons all-purpose flour
- 1 teaspoon baking soda
- 1 teaspoon salt
- 1 3/4 cups buttermilk
- 1 large egg
- 1 tablespoon vegetable shortening
- 1 tablespoon bacon grease

Direction

- Preheat oven to 475 degrees F.
- In a mixing bowl, combine the dry ingredients and mix well.
- In another bowl, combine the buttermilk and egg and beat till well blended, then add it to the dry ingredients and mix the batter till blended thoroughly.
- Place the shortening and bacon grease in a 9" iron skillet and heat till the shortening melts.
- Pour the hot fats into the batter, stir well, and pour the batter back into the skillet.
- Bake in the oven till the cornbread is golden brown, about 20 minutes.
- To serve, turn the skillet upside down on a big plate, remove, and cut the cornbread into wedges.
- (To prepare for Cornbread dressing, cool, cut into wedges and freeze until ready to use in recipe. Defrost before continuing.).

Nutrition Information

- Calories: 304.1
- Total Fat: 10.2
- Saturated Fat: 3.4
- Sugar: 5.5
- Cholesterol: 53.9
- Protein: 9.4
- Sodium: 1047.3
- Fiber: 3.5
- Total Carbohydrate: 44.7

311. Skinny Banana Blueberry Muffins

Serving: 12 muffins, 12 serving(s) | Prep: 10mins | Ready in:

Ingredients

- 2 1/2 cups white whole wheat flour (or mix of whole wheat and all-purpose)
- 1 teaspoon baking soda
- 1/4 teaspoon salt
- 1/2 teaspoon ground cinnamon
- 1/4 cup honey
- 1/2 cup light brown sugar, loosely packed (or dark brown sugar)
- 1 cup banana, mashed very ripe (about 2 large very ripe bananas)
- 1/4 cup nonfat yogurt, vanilla greek (or any yogurt)
- 1 large egg, beaten
- 3/4 cup milk (almond milk, soymilk, cow's milk, rice milk)
- 1 1/4 cups blueberries, fresh or 1 1/4 cups blueberries, frozen

Direction

- Preheat oven to 325F degrees. Spray 15 muffin tins with non-stick spray.* Set aside.
- In a large bowl, gently toss the flour, baking soda, salt, and cinnamon together until combined. Set aside.
- In a separate bowl, mix the honey and brown sugar together - it will be thick and lumpy. Try to get out as many lumps as you can - a fork works well to break it up. Add the mashed banana, yogurt, and beaten egg. Slowly pour the wet ingredients into the dry ingredients. Gently begin to fold it all together. It will be very thick. Add the milk slowly and continue

to gently mix the ingredients together. The milk will thin everything out, but the batter will still remain thick. Gently fold in the blueberries. Do not overmix the batter, which will lend tough, dry muffins.
- Divide the batter between 12 muffin tins. Fill all the way to the top. Bake for 20 minutes until very lightly browned on the edges. A toothpick inserted in the centre should come out clean. Allow the muffins to cool completely.
- *Note: Do not use cupcake liners; muffins will stick to them.

Nutrition Information

- Calories: 180.1
- Sodium: 174.3
- Total Carbohydrate: 39.1
- Cholesterol: 17.7
- Protein: 4.9
- Total Fat: 1.7
- Saturated Fat: 0.6
- Fiber: 3.4
- Sugar: 18.3

312. Snickerdoodle Muffins

Serving: 24 muffins | Prep: 15mins | Ready in:

Ingredients

- TOPPING
- 1/3 cup granulated sugar
- 1 teaspoon ground cinnamon
- MUFFIN
- 1 cup all-purpose flour
- 1/2 cup whole wheat flour
- 1 cup oats (quick or old fashioned, uncooked)
- 1/2 cup granulated sugar
- 1 tablespoon baking powder
- 1 cup nonfat milk
- 1 egg, lightly beaten
- 4 tablespoons margarine or 4 tablespoons butter, melted
- 1 teaspoon vanilla

Direction

- Heat oven to 400 degrees F. Spray bottoms only of mini muffin pan cups with cooking spray.
- For topping, combine sugar and cinnamon in small bowl; mix well and set aside.
- For muffins, combine flour, oats, sugar and baking powder in large bowl; mix well. In small bowl, combine milk, egg, margarine and vanilla; blend well. Add to dry ingredients all at once; stir just until dry ingredients are moistened. (Do not over mix.)
- Fill muffin cups two-thirds full. Sprinkle topping evenly over tops of muffins.
- Bake 12 to 14 minutes or until light golden brown. Cool muffins in pan on wire rack 5 minutes; remove from pan. Serve warm.

Nutrition Information

- Calories: 104
- Sodium: 75.2
- Fiber: 1.2
- Sugar: 7.5
- Cholesterol: 8
- Total Fat: 2.7
- Saturated Fat: 0.6
- Total Carbohydrate: 17.8
- Protein: 2.6

313. Souper Cornbread

Serving: 6-8 serving(s) | Prep: 10mins | Ready in:

Ingredients

- 1 (8 ounce) packagehouse-autry sweet yellow cornbread mix
- 1 (14 ounce) can cream-style corn, divided

Direction

- Preheat oven to 425°F.
- In a medium bowl, add the cornbread mix, but where the mix says to add 3/4 cup milk or water, instead substitute 3/4~1 cup of the creamed corn (start with 3/4 cup, then adjust for consistency). You want it to be moist enough where it practically pours into the pan.
- Bake in a greased 9" round cake pan for 11~14 minutes, or until golden brown and a toothpick inserted in the middle comes out clean.

Nutrition Information

- Calories: 205.9
- Saturated Fat: 1.2
- Fiber: 3.3
- Cholesterol: 0.8
- Total Fat: 4.9
- Total Carbohydrate: 38.3
- Protein: 3.8
- Sodium: 498.1
- Sugar: 9.8

314. Southern Biscuits

Serving: 10 serving(s) | Prep: 15mins | Ready in:

Ingredients

- 2 1/2 cups self rising flour
- 1/2-2/3 cup shortening
- 1 1/2-2 cups buttermilk

Direction

- Mix flour and shortening in a mixing bowl.
- Using a pastry blender or a fork, cut in shortening until mixture resembles coarse crumbs.
- Add buttermilk and stir.
- Start out with a little and add more as you need.
- The dough should be wet and gummy.
- THEN, sprinkle a little flour on top and work it in with your hands.
- Then flip the dough and do the same on the other side. Continue to do this until the dough isn't sticky on the outside, it doesn't take much.
- Then flour your hands and take a small amount of dough and roll it into a ball, then place on a greased cookie sheet or baking pan and flatten slightly into a biscuit shape. When you've finished with the dough, bake the biscuits in a 400 degree oven for about 10 minutes, just until they start to brown, then take them out and preheat the broiler, and then stick the biscuits back in until they are brown.
- You can brush them with melted butter if you like. This may take some practice, but after a few times you will know what the consistency of the dough should feel like. I hope this works for you.

Nutrition Information

- Calories: 215.9
- Saturated Fat: 2.8
- Sodium: 435.5
- Fiber: 0.8
- Total Carbohydrate: 24.9
- Protein: 4.3
- Total Fat: 10.9
- Sugar: 1.8
- Cholesterol: 1.5

315. Southern Cornbread Muffins

Serving: 12 serving(s) | Prep: 5mins | Ready in:

Ingredients

- 2 cups cornmeal
- 1/2 cup all-purpose flour

- 2 tablespoons sugar
- 1 teaspoon salt
- 1 teaspoon baking soda
- 1 3/4 cups buttermilk
- 1 egg, beaten
- 2 tablespoons butter or 2 tablespoons margarine, melted

Direction

- Combine cornmeal, flour, sugar, salt, and baking soda in a large bowl, mixing well.
- Combine buttermilk, egg, and butter, mixing well.
- Add to dry ingredients stirring just until moistened.
- Spoon into greased muffin pans. Bake at 425 for 15 minutes or until edges begin to brown.
- Yield is 1 dozen regular muffins or 6 Texas sized.

Nutrition Information

- Calories: 138.1
- Protein: 3.9
- Saturated Fat: 1.6
- Fiber: 1.6
- Sugar: 4
- Total Fat: 3.4
- Sodium: 362.9
- Total Carbohydrate: 23.4
- Cholesterol: 24.1

316. Southwest Biscuits

Serving: 20 serving(s) | Prep: 10mins | Ready in:

Ingredients

- 3 1/2 cups pancake mix
- 1 tablespoon taco seasoning mix
- 1 (10 ounce) candied tomatoes and chilies
- 1 cup milk
- 1 cup grated Mexican blend cheese

Direction

- Preheat oven to 425.
- In bowl, combine pancake mix and seasoning. Stir in tomatoes and chiles and milk.
- Fold in cheese. Use 2 tablespoon size scoop to drop dough onto baking sheets.
- Bake 11-14 minutes until golden.

Nutrition Information

- Calories: 123.9
- Saturated Fat: 1.8
- Sodium: 368.7
- Total Carbohydrate: 18.5
- Protein: 4.4
- Total Fat: 3.6
- Fiber: 0.8
- Sugar: 1.1
- Cholesterol: 13.4

317. Special Banana Blueberry Muffins

Serving: 12 muffins, 12 serving(s) | Prep: 15mins | Ready in:

Ingredients

- 2 cups flour
- 2 teaspoons baking powder
- 1/4 teaspoon baking soda
- 50 g butter, melted
- 1/2 cup sugar
- 1 large ripe banana, mashed
- 1/2 teaspoon vanilla
- 2 eggs
- 1/2 cup milk
- 1 orange, juice and rind of (1/2 cup juice)
- 1 cup blueberries (fresh or frozen)
- cinnamon sugar (use 3 tablespoons)
- 1/4 cup brown sugar
- 1/4 cup white sugar
- 1 tablespoon cinnamon

Direction

- Mix flour, baking powder and baking soda together in a large bowl.
- In another add the melted butter, then add the sugar, mashed banana, vanilla, eggs, milk, orange juice and rind.
- Mix with a fork to combine.
- Tip into dry ingredients and fold together until dry ingredients are barely damp.
- Stir in the (thawed) blueberries, taking care not to overmix.
- Spoon mixture into deep, buttered or sprayed muffin pans and sprinkle each muffin with 1/4 tsp cinnamon sugar.
- Bake at 200 degrees for 10-12 minutes or until muffins spring back when pressed in centre.

Nutrition Information

- Calories: 214.4
- Sodium: 129.8
- Fiber: 1.7
- Total Carbohydrate: 39.7
- Cholesterol: 45.6
- Total Fat: 4.9
- Saturated Fat: 2.7
- Sugar: 20.7
- Protein: 3.9

318. Spicy Orange Bran Muffins

Serving: 12 serving(s) | Prep: 10mins | Ready in:

Ingredients

- 1 1/2 cups natural bran
- 1 3/4 cups buttermilk
- 1 1/4 cups whole wheat flour
- 1 teaspoon baking powder
- 1/2 teaspoon baking soda
- 2 teaspoons cinnamon
- 1/2 cup raisins
- 2 tablespoons orange zest
- 1 egg
- 1/4 cup brown sugar, loosely packed
- 1/4 cup canola oil
- 2 tablespoons molasses
- 2 tablespoons honey

Direction

- Combine bran and buttermilk, let stand while assembling other ingredients.
- In bowl, combine remaining dry ingredients.
- In another bowl, combine egg, brown sugar, honey, molasses and oil.
- Mix well.
- Add bran mixture.
- Add dry ingredients.
- Bake in sprayed muffin tin in 375 degree oven for 20 minutes.
- Best served warm.

Nutrition Information

- Calories: 180.2
- Saturated Fat: 0.7
- Fiber: 4.3
- Sugar: 15.7
- Total Carbohydrate: 31.6
- Protein: 4.6
- Total Fat: 5.9
- Sodium: 148.8
- Cholesterol: 19.1

319. Strawberry Banana Wheat And Oat Muffins

Serving: 12 muffins, 12 serving(s) | Prep: 10mins | Ready in:

Ingredients

- 1 1/2 cups wheat flour
- 1 cup oatmeal
- 1/2 cup sugar

- 2 teaspoons baking powder
- 2 bananas, mashed
- 1 teaspoon vanilla
- 1/2 cup skim milk
- 1/4 cup egg substitute
- 2 tablespoons olive oil
- 1 cup frozen strawberries, diced

Direction

- Preheat oven to 375.
- Mix all dry ingredients in a medium bowl and set aside.
- Mix all wet ingredients and combine with the dry.
- Spray a 12 hole muffin pan with cooking spray, (I prefer the one with flour).
- Fill muffins 3/4 full and place in oven for 17 minutes.

Nutrition Information

- Calories: 162.8
- Protein: 4.5
- Saturated Fat: 0.5
- Fiber: 3.4
- Total Carbohydrate: 30.8
- Cholesterol: 0.3
- Total Fat: 3.2
- Sodium: 77.5
- Sugar: 11.8

320. Strawberry And Cream Cheese Filled Muffins

Serving: 12 serving(s) | Prep: 20mins | Ready in:

Ingredients

- 1/4 cup reduced-fat cream cheese
- 2 tablespoons strawberry preserves
- 2 1/4 cups flour
- 1/3 cup sugar
- 2 teaspoons baking powder
- 2 teaspoons poppy seeds
- 1/2 teaspoon baking soda
- 1/4 teaspoon salt
- 1 1/4 cups low-fat buttermilk
- 3 tablespoons vegetable oil
- 2 large egg whites
- 1 large egg

Direction

- Preheat oven to 375°.
- Combine the cream cheese and preserves; stir with a whisk.
- Lightly spoon flour into dry measuring cups; level with a knife.
- Combine flour, sugar, baking powder, poppy seeds, baking soda and salt in a medium bowl; make a well in center of mixture.
- Combine buttermilk, oil, egg whites, and egg; stir well with a whisk.
- Add to flour mixture, stirring just until moist.
- Spoon the batter into 12 muffin cups coated with cooking spray, filling one-third full.
- Top each with about 1 teaspoon cream cheese mixture, divide the remaining batter evenly over the cream cheese mixture.
- Bake at 375° for 25 minutes or until muffins spring back when touched lightly in center.
- Remove the muffins from pans immediately, and place on a wire rack.

Nutrition Information

- Calories: 179.6
- Sugar: 8.6
- Total Carbohydrate: 27.6
- Total Fat: 5.4
- Saturated Fat: 1.3
- Sodium: 219.6
- Fiber: 0.7
- Cholesterol: 21.4
- Protein: 5

321. Strawberry Orange Muffins!!!

Serving: 12 muffins | Prep: 10mins | Ready in:

Ingredients

- 1 1/4 cups halved strawberries
- 3 tablespoons butter, melted
- 2 teaspoons grated orange rind
- 2 large eggs
- 1 1/2 cups all-purpose flour
- 1 1/4 cups sugar
- 1 teaspoon baking powder
- 1/2 teaspoon salt
- cooking spray
- 2 teaspoons sugar
- jam or preserves

Direction

- Preheat oven to 400
- Combine the first 4 ingredients in a blender and process just until mixture is blended.
- Lightly spoon flour into dry measuring cups and level with a knife.
- Combine flour, 1 1/4 cups sugar, baking powder, and salt.
- Add strawberry mixture to flour mixture stirring just until mixture is moist.
- Spoon batter into 12 muffin cups coated with cooking spray.
- Sprinkle batter evenly with 2 teaspoons sugar.
- Bake at 400 for 20 minutes or until muffins spring back when touched lightly in center.
- Remove muffins from pan immediately and serve with jam if desired.
- ** NOTE: set timer for 15 minutes because muffins tend to cook fast.

Nutrition Information

- Calories: 183.2
- Total Fat: 3.9
- Saturated Fat: 2.1
- Sodium: 159.7
- Fiber: 0.8
- Sugar: 22.3
- Total Carbohydrate: 34.9
- Cholesterol: 42.9
- Protein: 2.8

322. Sue's Rice Muffins

Serving: 6 muffins, 6 serving(s) | Prep: 5mins | Ready in:

Ingredients

- 1 egg
- 1/2 cup water
- 1/2 cup unsweetened applesauce
- 2 tablespoons canola oil
- 1 cup rice flour
- 2 teaspoons baking powder

Direction

- Preheat oven to 425 degrees F. Lightly grease a 6 cup muffin tin, set aside.
- In a one quart jar place all ingredients; mix well. Pour into prepared muffin tin.
- Bake for 17 - 20 minutes. Allow muffins to cool for 5-8 minutes before removing from tin.
- Yield: 6 muffins.

Nutrition Information

- Calories: 159.4
- Sodium: 133.5
- Fiber: 0.9
- Sugar: 0.1
- Total Carbohydrate: 23.8
- Cholesterol: 35.2
- Protein: 2.6
- Saturated Fat: 0.7
- Total Fat: 5.9

323. Sugar Free Cinnamon Raisin Muffins

Serving: 12 serving(s) | Prep: 10mins | Ready in:

Ingredients

- 4 tablespoons light margarine, melted
- 1 cup unsweetened applesauce
- 2 egg whites
- 4 ounces plain fat-free yogurt, plain
- 1/4 cup Splenda granular, sugar substitute or 1/4 cup honey
- 1 3/4 cups dry quick oats
- 1/3 cup millet
- 1/2 cup brown rice flour
- 1 tablespoon vanilla extract
- 1 teaspoon baking soda
- 1 teaspoon baking powder
- 1 tablespoon ground cinnamon
- 3/4 cup raisins

Direction

- Mix the first five ingredients.
- Add dry ingredients and raisins.
- Mix well.
- Bake at 350 degrees for about 15 minutes or until toothpick pulls out clean.

Nutrition Information

- Calories: 139
- Saturated Fat: 0.2
- Sodium: 154.4
- Fiber: 2.8
- Total Carbohydrate: 27.9
- Cholesterol: 0.2
- Sugar: 6.5
- Protein: 4.5
- Total Fat: 1.3

324. Sumner's Favorite Healthy Rhubarb Scones

Serving: 8 scones, 8 serving(s) | Prep: 15mins | Ready in:

Ingredients

- 1 1/2 cups all-purpose flour
- 1 cup whole wheat flour
- 1/2 cup sugar
- 2 1/2 teaspoons baking powder
- 1/2 teaspoon baking soda
- 1/2 teaspoon salt
- 1/2 cup low-fat buttermilk
- 1/2 cup skim milk
- 1 egg
- 2 stalks rhubarb

Direction

- Line baking sheet with parchment paper and preheat oven to 400.
- In bowl whisk together flour, sugar, baking powder, baking soda and salt.
- In small bowl whisk buttermilk with egg. Drizzle over dry ingredients and stir together with a fork. (Dough should be very sticky) Knead in the rhubarb.
- Pat into a ball with your hands. Cut into 8 triangles and place each one onto the baking sheet.
- Bake in the center of the oven for 12-15 minutes. Let cool on rack. Keep in airtight container.

Nutrition Information

- Calories: 209.5
- Saturated Fat: 0.4
- Fiber: 2.5
- Sugar: 13.5
- Cholesterol: 24.2
- Protein: 6.4
- Total Fat: 1.4
- Sodium: 372.9
- Total Carbohydrate: 43.7

325. Sun Dried Tomato Biscuits

Serving: 12 biscuits. | Prep: 15mins | Ready in:

Ingredients

- 2 cups unbleached white flour
- 1 tablespoon baking powder
- 1 tablespoon granulated sugar
- 1 teaspoon salt
- 1/2 cup unsalted butter, frozen
- 2 eggs
- 1/2 cup buttermilk
- 1/3 cup sun-dried tomato, finely chopped
- 1 tablespoon finely chopped thyme

Direction

- Preheat oven to 400 degrees. In a large bowl, sift together the dry ingredients. Finely chop the butter. By hand or in a food processor, blend with the dry ingredients. The mixture should not be thoroughly blended, but should have small, pea-sized clumps of butter and flour. In a small bowl, whisk the eggs and buttermilk together. Stir in the sun-dried tomatoes and thyme. Work together the dry and moist ingredients until the dough begins to come together. Do not overwork or your biscuits will be tough. Turn the dough onto a floured board and roll into 1/2-inch thickness. Fold in half and roll out again. Fold in half one more time and roll into 3/4-inch thickness. Cut the dough into 2-inch square biscuits. Bake on a lightly oiled baking sheet for about 12 minutes or until the biscuits are fluffy and browned.
- Makes about 12 biscuits.

Nutrition Information

- Calories: 168.6
- Sodium: 339.8
- Sugar: 2.2
- Protein: 3.8
- Total Fat: 8.8
- Saturated Fat: 5.2
- Fiber: 0.8
- Total Carbohydrate: 18.6
- Cholesterol: 56

326. Super Fast Easy Onion Cheese Muffins

Serving: 12 muffins, 12 serving(s) | Prep: 5mins | Ready in:

Ingredients

- 3 cups Bisquick
- 1 teaspoon salt
- 3/4 cup cheddar cheese, shredded
- 1 (3 1/2 ounce) can French-fried onions, crumbled
- 1 egg
- 1 cup milk

Direction

- Combine all ingredients in a large bowl. Beat 1 minute. Fill muffin tins (greased) 2/3 full. Bake at 400* for about 15 minutes.

Nutrition Information

- Calories: 176
- Total Fat: 8.1
- Saturated Fat: 3.3
- Sugar: 3.6
- Protein: 5.3
- Sodium: 636.2
- Fiber: 0.6
- Total Carbohydrate: 20.1
- Cholesterol: 28.5

327. Super Simple Cranberry Coconut Scones

Serving: 12-15 serving(s) | Prep: 5mins | Ready in:

Ingredients

- 1 (8 ounce) boxjiffy biscuit mix
- 2/3 cup heavy whipping cream
- 1 cup coconut
- 1/4 cup sugar
- 1/2 teaspoon cinnamon
- 1/8 teaspoon ginger
- 1/8 teaspoon nutmeg
- 1 teaspoon orange rind
- 1/4 cup craisins (orange-flavored dried cranberries)
- 1/2 cup coarsely chopped pecans

Direction

- Mix together all dry ingredients.
- Add the cream and mix just until all ingredients are moistened.
- Drop by tablespoonfuls on a lightly greased baking sheet.
- Sprinkle the mounds of dough lightly with sugar.
- Bake 15 minutes in a 375 degree oven.
- Remove immediately to cooling rack.

Nutrition Information

- Calories: 229.1
- Saturated Fat: 8.1
- Cholesterol: 18.5
- Sodium: 248.9
- Fiber: 2.2
- Sugar: 8.7
- Total Carbohydrate: 21
- Protein: 2.7
- Total Fat: 15.7

328. Super Moist Cornbread

Serving: 8 serving(s) | Prep: 5mins | Ready in:

Ingredients

- 1 (11 ounce) can Mexican-style corn, drained
- 1 (8 1/2 ounce) package corn muffin mix
- 1/2 cup mayonnaise (Hellmann's or Best Foods)
- 1 egg, slightly beaten

Direction

- Preheat oven to 400 degrees F. Spray 8-inch round cake pan with nonstick-cooking spray; set aside.
- In medium bowl, combine all ingredients until moistened. Spread evenly in prepared pan.
- Bake 25 minutes or until toothpick inserted in center comes out clean.

Nutrition Information

- Calories: 221.6
- Saturated Fat: 1.9
- Fiber: 2
- Sugar: 7.1
- Total Carbohydrate: 31.6
- Protein: 3.9
- Total Fat: 9.4
- Sodium: 583.1
- Cholesterol: 30.9

329. Sweet And Nutty Raisin Bran Muffins

Serving: 12 serving(s) | Prep: 15mins | Ready in:

Ingredients

- 1 cup applesauce
- 3/4 cup brown sugar
- 1/4 cup Dark Karo syrup or 1/4 cup molasses or 1/4 cup maple syrup

- 2 egg whites (whipped until peaks form)
- 1 cup all-purpose flour
- 1 teaspoon baking powder
- 1/2 teaspoon salt
- 1/2 teaspoon baking soda
- 1 teaspoon cinnamon or 1 teaspoon nutmeg
- 2 cups Raisin Bran cereal
- Topping
- 1/2 cup brown sugar
- 1/2 cup crushed pecans

Direction

- Sift together dry ingredients except for the cereal.
- Mix applesauce, sugar, syrup together.
- Add the flour mixture to the syrup mixture.
- Next add cereal.
- Last fold in the egg whites.
- Spoon batter into a lightly greased or sprayed muffin pan (12 count muffin tin).
- Mix together the sugar and the pecans.
- Sprinkle topping on to the batter.
- Bake muffins in a 400° preheated oven for 15-20 minutes.
- Let cool or serve hot with sweet Honey Butter, or just plain, their great!

Nutrition Information

- Calories: 227.4
- Fiber: 2.3
- Sugar: 27.4
- Protein: 3
- Total Fat: 3.7
- Total Carbohydrate: 48.5
- Cholesterol: 0
- Saturated Fat: 0.4
- Sodium: 274.8

330. The Best Peach Nectarine Muffins

Serving: 8 serving(s) | Prep: 10mins | Ready in:

Ingredients

- 1 1/2 cups flour
- 3/4 cup white sugar
- 1/2 teaspoon salt
- 2 teaspoons baking powder
- 1/3 cup vegetable oil
- 1 egg
- 1/3 cup milk
- 1 ripe peach (peeled, pitted, and diced)
- 1 ripe nectarine, pitted and diced (or use 1 1/2 cup other fruit)
- 1/8-1/4 cup brown sugar

Direction

- Preheat oven to 400 degrees.
- Grease 8 muffin cups or use paper liners.
- In a large bowl combine flour, white sugar, salt, and baking powder.
- Add oil, egg, and milk.
- Stir only until blended together.
- Fold in fruit.
- Fill muffin tins to the top.
- Sprinkle tops with brown sugar.
- Bake 15-20 minutes.

Nutrition Information

- Calories: 282.3
- Total Fat: 10.4
- Saturated Fat: 1.6
- Cholesterol: 24.7
- Protein: 3.9
- Sodium: 251.6
- Fiber: 1.2
- Sugar: 25.1
- Total Carbohydrate: 44.5

331. The Realtor's Cheesy Pepper Scones

Serving: 12 serving(s) | Prep: 5mins | Ready in:

Ingredients

- 6 tablespoons butter, divided use
- 1 onion, finely chopped
- 1/2 cup chopped red bell pepper
- 2 cups all-purpose flour
- 1 tablespoon baking powder
- 1/2 teaspoon salt
- 1/4 teaspoon white pepper
- 1/4 teaspoon ground cayenne pepper
- 1 cup shredded gruyere cheese (can sub Monterey Jack)
- 1/2 cup shredded cheddar cheese
- 3/4 cup milk

Direction

- Preheat oven to 425*F.
- Melt 2 tablespoons butter in a skillet and sauté chopped onion and chopped red bell pepper until soft; set aside.
- In a large bowl mix together flour, baking powder, salt, white pepper, and cayenne pepper. Cut in 4 tablespoons butter until coarse crumbs are formed. Stir in Gruyere cheese, cheddar cheese, the onion mixture, and milk; stir just to blend.
- On a lightly floured flat surface, form the dough into 12 rounds, flatten, and place on a greased baking sheet. Brush with milk. Bake for 15 minutes.

Nutrition Information

- Calories: 180
- Cholesterol: 27.3
- Saturated Fat: 5.7
- Total Carbohydrate: 18.3
- Sugar: 0.8
- Protein: 5.5
- Total Fat: 9.5
- Sodium: 267.1
- Fiber: 0.8

332. The Ruby Pear Tea Parlor's Cinnamon Chip Scones

Serving: 30 scones | Prep: 15mins | Ready in:

Ingredients

- 6 cups self rising flour
- 3/4 cup sugar
- 1 cup butter, room temperature
- 2 cups cinnamon baking chips
- 2 cups evaporated milk

Direction

- 1. Preheat oven to 350 degrees.
- 2. Combine flour and sugar. Cut in the butter. Add cinnamon chips and mix well. Add the evaporated milk and mix well to form dough.
- 3. Turn out onto a floured surface. Knead lightly and pat out to 1/2 inch thickness. Cut out 2 inch scone portions.
- 4. Bake for 13 minutes.

Nutrition Information

- Calories: 184.6
- Total Fat: 7.7
- Fiber: 0.7
- Total Carbohydrate: 25.2
- Saturated Fat: 4.7
- Sodium: 389.4
- Sugar: 5
- Cholesterol: 21.1
- Protein: 3.7

333. Three Cheese Onion Muffins

Serving: 12 serving(s) | Prep: 10mins | Ready in:

Ingredients

- 2 cups all-purpose flour
- 3 teaspoons baking powder
- 1/4 teaspoon pepper
- 1 dash ground nutmeg
- 1 1/4 cups milk
- 1/4 cup butter or 1/4 cup margarine, melted
- 1 egg
- 1/4 cup chopped green onion
- 1/4 cup shredded mozzarella cheese
- 1/4 cup grated romano cheese
- 1/4 cup shredded parmesan cheese

Direction

- Preheat oven to 400 degrees.
- In a bowl, combine the flour, baking powder, pepper and nutmeg.
- In another bowl, combine the milk, butter and egg.
- Combine wet and dry ingredients and stir only until moistened.
- Fold in the onions and cheeses.
- Fill greased muffin cups two-thirds full.
- Bake 16-18 minutes, or until toothpick inserted in center of muffin comes out clean.
- Cool 5 minutes before removing from pan to wire rack.

Nutrition Information

- Calories: 156.2
- Saturated Fat: 4.2
- Sodium: 211.4
- Fiber: 0.6
- Sugar: 0.2
- Total Fat: 7
- Total Carbohydrate: 17.8
- Cholesterol: 34.8
- Protein: 5.5

334. Thunder Bay Grille Biscuits

Serving: 12 biscuits, 12 serving(s) | Prep: 5mins | Ready in:

Ingredients

- 2 1/2 cups flour
- 1/2 cup sugar
- 1/8 cup sugar
- 2 tablespoons baking powder
- 1/4 teaspoon salt
- 1/3 cup margarine or 1/3 cup softened butter
- 1 1/8 cups milk

Direction

- Stir together flour, both measures of sugar, baking powder and salt in a large mixing bowl.
- Blend in margarine or butter until the mixture is crumbly.
- Add milk a little at a time and mix to make a stiff dough. You might not use all of the milk.
- Drop by heaping tablespoons onto a greased cookie sheet.
- Bake at 370 degrees until golden brown, approximately 12 minutes.
- CINNAMON BUTTER.
- 1 stick soft butter.
- 1/8 cup brown sugar.
- 3/4 teaspoon cinnamon.
- Dash of vanilla.
- Whip all ingredients together with a mixer or wire whip until well blended. Serve with Thunder Bay Biscuits, alongside quick breads or muffins, or over French toast or pancakes!

Nutrition Information

- Calories: 173.5
- Sodium: 271.4

- Fiber: 0.7
- Total Carbohydrate: 31.9
- Protein: 3.5
- Total Fat: 3.6
- Saturated Fat: 1.1
- Cholesterol: 3.2
- Sugar: 10.5

335. Tims' Mom's Blueberry Muffins

Serving: 12 muffins, 12 serving(s) | Prep: 5mins | Ready in:

Ingredients

- 1 3/4 cups all-purpose flour (White Lily)
- 2/3 cup sugar
- 1 tablespoon baking powder
- 1 teaspoon salt
- 8 tablespoons butter (1 stick)
- 1 egg, sightly beaten
- 1 teaspoon grated lemons, rind of or 1 tablespoon lemon juice
- 1 teaspoon vanilla
- 1/2 cup milk
- 2 tablespoons vegetable oil
- 1 cup blueberries, if frozen, do not thaw

Direction

- Cut butter into flour, sugar, baking powder and salt.
- (Like you do for pie crust) Add egg, lemon, milk vegetable oil and vanilla, stir just till moist fold in blueberries.
- Bake in well-greased muffin tin at 400 degrees for 20 to 25 minutes.
- Muffin cups will be about 2/3 full.

Nutrition Information

- Calories: 218.7
- Sodium: 363.7

- Fiber: 0.8
- Total Carbohydrate: 27.7
- Protein: 2.9
- Saturated Fat: 5.5
- Cholesterol: 37.3
- Total Fat: 10.9
- Sugar: 12.5

336. Toasted English Muffins With Cheese

Serving: 12 serving(s) | Prep: 10mins | Ready in:

Ingredients

- 6 English muffins, cut in half and toasted
- 1 cup cheddar cheese, grated
- 1 cup mayonnaise
- 1 1/2 teaspoons curry powder
- 1/4 cup chopped green olives
- 1/4 cup green onion, chopped (optional)

Direction

- Mix the cheddar cheese, mayonnaise, curry powder, olives and green onion, if using, together.
- Spread on toasted muffins; put in the oven at 350°F for 8-10 minutes.

Nutrition Information

- Calories: 183.9
- Total Fat: 10.6
- Saturated Fat: 3.2
- Sodium: 344.6
- Fiber: 1.2
- Total Carbohydrate: 17.6
- Sugar: 2.3
- Cholesterol: 15
- Protein: 5.1

337. Uncle Bill's Yorkshire Pudding

Serving: 12 muffins | Prep: 10mins | Ready in:

Ingredients

- 1 cup whole milk, homogenized
- 1 cup all-purpose flour
- 3 large eggs
- 1/2 teaspoon salt
- 18 teaspoons extra virgin olive oil

Direction

- Preheat oven to 450 degrees F.
- In a mixing bowl, combine milk and flour.
- Add eggs one at a time and beat well after each addition until batter is smooth.
- Add salt and mix well.
- Heat a 12 cup muffin pan for 3 minutes in preheated 450 F oven.
- Remove pan from oven and add 1 1/2 teaspoons of olive oil to each muffin cup.
- Return muffin pan to preheated 450 F oven and heat for about 2 minutes or until oil gets hot (THIS IS VERY IMPORANT.) Remove heated pan from oven and spoon about 3 tablespoons of batter into each cup until mixture is evenly distributed in the 12 cups.
- Return to oven and bake in preheated 450 F oven for 10 minutes.
- Reduce heat to 350 F and continue to bake for another 10 minutes or until Yorkshire pudding has risen and is lightly browned.
- DO NOT OPEN OVEN DOOR AT ANYTIME DURING THE BAKING PERIOD.
- At the end of the baking time specified, you may open the oven door to take a peek at the pudding to see if it has risen and is lightly browned.
- Remove from oven and serve immediately with your favorite gravy recipe along with your roast.
- If you have any fat from your roast, you may use this in lieu of the olive oil.
- Prepare muffin pan in the same manner.
- For an easy gravy, see recipe #25365.

Nutrition Information

- Calories: 127.9
- Protein: 3.3
- Saturated Fat: 1.7
- Cholesterol: 48.5
- Total Carbohydrate: 9
- Total Fat: 8.7
- Sodium: 123.7
- Fiber: 0.3
- Sugar: 1.1

338. Vanilla Freezer Biscuits (Cookies) (With Variations)

Serving: 40 biscuits/cookies, 40 serving(s) | Prep: 15mins | Ready in:

Ingredients

- 1 vanilla bean (halved lengthways)
- 250 g butter (softened)
- 1 cup caster sugar
- 1 egg
- 2 1/2 cups plain flour
- 4 tablespoons powdered sugar icing (to serve)

Direction

- Scrape seeds from vanilla bean (they advise you discard the bean but stick it in a canister of sugar and you will soon have vanilla sugar).
- Beat butter, sugar and bean seeds until pale and creamy using an electric mixer.
- Add egg and beat until combined.
- Sift flour over butter mixture and use a wooden spoon, stir to combine.
- Place dough on a lightly floured surface and divide in half.
- Using hands shape each half in a 30cm long log.

- Wrap each log in baking paper, twirling ends to seal.
- Freeze for 2 hours or until firm.
- Remove logs from freezer 15 minutes before slicing.
- Preheat oven to 180 degree C (160 C for fan forced).
- Line 2 baking trays with baking paper.
- Remove paper from logs and slice into 1.5cm thick rounds.
- Place rounds, 3cm apart on prepared trays.
- Bake for 12 to 14 minutes or until light golden colour.
- Cool on trays for 5 minutes and transfer to wire rack to cool completely.
- Dust with icing sugar and serve.
- You can leave logs in freezer for up to 2 months, thaw for 1 hour before slicing and baking.
- VARIATIONS.
- Chocolate chips - Stir 1/2 cup chopped dark chocolate chips at the end of step 4.
- Pistachio - Stir in 2/3 cups of roughly chopped pistachio kernels at the end of step 4.
- Citrus - Add 1 tablespoon finely grated lemon or orange rind with vanilla bean seeds in step 2.

Nutrition Information

- Calories: 94.1
- Saturated Fat: 3.2
- Sugar: 5
- Total Carbohydrate: 11
- Cholesterol: 18
- Protein: 1
- Total Fat: 5.2
- Sodium: 46.3
- Fiber: 0.2

339. Vanilla Muffins

Serving: 10-12 serving(s) | Prep: 15mins | Ready in:

Ingredients

- 1 cup sugar
- 1 egg, beaten
- 2 cups flour
- 2 teaspoons baking powder
- 1 cup milk
- 1/4 cup melted butter
- 2 1/2 teaspoons vanilla
- 1 1/2 teaspoons sugar
- 1/8 teaspoon cinnamon

Direction

- Combine sugar and egg, beat well. Combine flour and baking powder. Add to sugar mixture, alternately with the milk, beginning and ending with the flour mixture, beating well after each addition. Stir in butter and vanilla. Spoon into greased muffin pans, filling 2/3 full.
- Combine sugar and cinnamon and sprinkle evenly over muffins.
- Bake at 375°F for 15-20 minutes.

Nutrition Information

- Calories: 237.9
- Saturated Fat: 3.7
- Sodium: 133
- Sugar: 20.8
- Cholesterol: 34.2
- Total Fat: 6.2
- Fiber: 0.7
- Total Carbohydrate: 41.3
- Protein: 4.1

340. Vegan Apple Muffins

Serving: 12 muffins, 12 serving(s) | Prep: 10mins | Ready in:

Ingredients

- 1 cup flour

- 3/4 cup whole wheat flour
- 3/4 cup quick-cooking oats
- 1 3/4 teaspoons baking powder
- 1 -2 teaspoon cinnamon
- 3/4 teaspoon baking soda
- 1/4 teaspoon salt
- 3/4 cup rice milk
- 3/4 cup canola oil
- 1 1/2 teaspoons Ener-G Egg Substitute, mixed with
- 2 tablespoons water
- 2/3 cup evaporated cane juice (or packed brown sugar)
- 1 teaspoon vanilla
- 1 apple, diced
- cinnamon sugar, for sprinkling the muffin tops (optional)

Direction

- Preheat oven to 375 and prepare 12 regular or 6 jumbo muffin cups with liners or non-stick baking spray.
- In large bowl, combine the flours, baking powder, cinnamon, baking soda, and salt.
- In separate bowl, stir together milk, oil, egg replacement, and vanilla.
- Make a well in the dry ingredients; pour wet ingredients over well.
- Add apple and stir until just moistened.
- Fill muffin cups 3/4 way full.
- Sprinkle tops of muffins with cinnamon sugar, if desired.
- Bake for 25 minutes. Let cool in pan for 5 minutes before removing.
- Will keep in airtight container for a couple of days, or in the freezer for 2-3 weeks.

Nutrition Information

- Calories: 218.6
- Fiber: 2.1
- Sugar: 1.4
- Total Carbohydrate: 20.3
- Cholesterol: 0
- Total Fat: 14.3
- Sodium: 186.4
- Protein: 3
- Saturated Fat: 1.1

341. Vegan Carrot Ginger Muffins

Serving: 7 serving(s) | Prep: 10mins | Ready in:

Ingredients

- 2 cups flour
- 1/2 cup sugar
- 1 teaspoon baking soda
- 1 teaspoon baking powder
- 1/2 teaspoon salt
- 1/2 teaspoon cinnamon
- 1 cup raisins
- 2 medium carrots, grated
- 3/4 cup soymilk
- 2 eggs, equivalent
- 2 tablespoons applesauce
- 2 tablespoons oil
- 2 tablespoons ginger, grated

Direction

- Preheat oven to 400 degrees.
- Mix dry ingredients.
- Add wet ingredients.
- Stir until combined.
- Bake for 12-15 minutes.

Nutrition Information

- Calories: 332.8
- Protein: 7.6
- Saturated Fat: 1.1
- Sugar: 27.7
- Total Carbohydrate: 63.3
- Fiber: 2.9
- Cholesterol: 60.4
- Total Fat: 6.4
- Sodium: 449

342. Vegan Fat Free Biscuits

Serving: 6 biscuits, 2 serving(s) | Prep: 10mins | Ready in:

Ingredients

- 1 cup oat flour (you can make it by whirring rolled oats in the food processor)
- 1/2 teaspoon baking soda (I live at high altitude, so you might need a bit more at sea level)
- 1/8 teaspoon salt
- 1/2 cup unsweetened applesauce

Direction

- Preheat oven to 400 F and coat a cookie sheet with a thin layer of oil.
- Whisk dry ingredients together, then stir in applesauce.
- Drop onto cookie sheet in biscuit size drops (should make 6 - they will be sticky).
- Bake 8 -10 mins until lightly brown.
- Smother in your favorite vegan gravy or top with jam. They are especially good topped with a spinach "cream" sauce. The oat flour makes them much more tender than wheat as there is no gluten.

Nutrition Information

- Calories: 226.6
- Total Fat: 1.9
- Saturated Fat: 0.4
- Cholesterol: 0
- Sodium: 467.8
- Fiber: 6.7
- Sugar: 7.3
- Total Carbohydrate: 49.2
- Protein: 7.7

343. Vegan Tomato Rosemary Scones (With Gluten Free Option)

Serving: 12 scones, 12 serving(s) | Prep: 10mins | Ready in:

Ingredients

- 3 cups all-purpose flour (OR Bob's Red Mill Gluten-Free All-Purpose Baking Flour plus 1 teaspoon xantham gum)
- 2 tablespoons baking powder
- 1/4 cup sugar
- 1/2 teaspoon salt
- 1/2 teaspoon ground black pepper
- 1/3 cup olive oil
- 1 (14 ounce) can tomato sauce (about 1 1/2 cups)
- 1 teaspoon apple cider vinegar
- 2 tablespoons fresh rosemary, chopped (about 4 sprigs)

Direction

- Preheat the oven to 400 degrees Fahrenheit. Lightly grease a large baking sheet.
- In a large mixing bowl, combine flour, baking powder, sugar, salt, and pepper.
- In another bowl, combine wet ingredients and rosemary.
- Make a well in the center of the dry ingredients and pour in the liquid. Gently mix with a wooden spoon.
- When the batter is loosely holding together, turn it onto a lightly floured work surface and gently knead until a soft dough forms. DO NOT overmix. Some patches of flour are good. Add a little extra flour if the dough seems sticky. Divide dough in two and form each section into a 6-inch disk. Slice each disk into six pieces (cut in half and then cut each half into thirds). OR if you are lazy like me and don't need your scones to be pretty, you can just scoop the dough into 8-12 mounds on the cookie sheet (like drop biscuits).

- Place scones on the baking sheet and bake 14-16 minutes or until the tops are firm. Remove and let cool a bit on plate or cooling rack. Serve either warm or at room temperature.

Nutrition Information

- Calories: 192.7
- Protein: 3.7
- Sodium: 454
- Sugar: 5.7
- Fiber: 1.4
- Total Carbohydrate: 30.5
- Cholesterol: 0
- Total Fat: 6.4
- Saturated Fat: 0.9

344. Vegetarian Pizza Muffins

Serving: 4 serving(s) | Prep: 10mins | Ready in:

Ingredients

- 1 cup ricotta cheese
- 1 cup mozzarella cheese or 1 cup swiss cheese, shredded
- 1/3 cup grated parmesan cheese
- 1/4 cup bottled roasted red pepper, chopped
- 1/2 teaspoon dried oregano
- 1 clove garlic, minced
- 4 whole wheat English muffins, split and toasted
- 10 ounces broccoli florets, thawed if frozen

Direction

- Preheat oven to 375 degrees.
- Combine first 6 ingredients in a bowl.
- Spread about 2 tablespoons on each muffin half and place on cookie sheet.
- Top with broccoli and remaining cheese mixture.
- Bake 10 minutes or until cheese melts.

Nutrition Information

- Calories: 385.8
- Fiber: 4.6
- Sugar: 5.9
- Total Fat: 18.3
- Sodium: 735.8
- Protein: 24.6
- Saturated Fat: 10.5
- Total Carbohydrate: 34.2
- Cholesterol: 60.8

345. Weight Watcher's Cheese Muffins

Serving: 12 small muffins | Prep: 5mins | Ready in:

Ingredients

- 1 1/2 cups self-raising flour
- 2 cups low-fat cheese, grated
- 1/2 teaspoon salt
- 1 tablespoon sugar
- 1 pinch cayenne
- 1 egg, slightly beaten
- 1 cup low-fat milk

Direction

- Preheat oven to 210C (or 350F) then spray muffin tin with spray-on oil.
- Mix together dry ingredients in a bowl.
- In another bowl mix wet ingredients. Add the wet ingredients to the dry ones. Do not over mix or it will be rubbery.
- Bake for about 12 minutes or until they spring back when touched.

Nutrition Information

- Calories: 74.2
- Total Carbohydrate: 13.7
- Cholesterol: 18.6
- Sugar: 2.2

- Saturated Fat: 0.3
- Sodium: 310.1
- Fiber: 0.4
- Protein: 2.8
- Total Fat: 0.8

346. Wheaten Scones (Diabetic Friendly)

Serving: 9 scones, 9 serving(s) | Prep: 15mins | Ready in:

Ingredients

- 225 g wholemeal flour
- 225 g all-purpose flour
- 1 teaspoon baking soda
- 1 teaspoon salt
- 25 g butter (optional)
- 250 ml buttermilk or 250 ml milk with 1 tablespoon lemon juice
- 1 egg, beaten

Direction

- Pre heat oven to 200/180 fan /gas 6
- Sieve flour, salt, baking soda in a bowl then add the w/w flour and mix well.
- Rub in butter if using.
- Make a well in middle and pour in the buttermilk egg mixture and mix quickly do not over mix it must be a soft mix.
- Roll out to 1 inch thick and cut out or you can cut into triangles.
- I brush with a bit of milk and top with a sprinkle of wheat bran.
- Bake in oven 15 to 20 minutes.
- Cool on a wire rack and cover with a clean tea towel.

Nutrition Information

- Calories: 201.3
- Saturated Fat: 0.4
- Sugar: 1.5

- Total Fat: 1.3
- Sodium: 436.9
- Fiber: 1.4
- Total Carbohydrate: 39.5
- Cholesterol: 21.8
- Protein: 6.8

347. Whipping Cream Biscuits

Serving: 3 dozen | Prep: 5mins | Ready in:

Ingredients

- 1 1/2 cups self rising flour
- 1/2 pint whipping cream

Direction

- Mix the flour and the cream until blended;
- Butter hands well and form the dough into ping pong ball sizes.
- Place on baking sheet 1 inch apart.
- Bake at 425°F for 10 to 12 minutes or until golden brown.

Nutrition Information

- Calories: 494.9
- Total Fat: 30
- Fiber: 1.7
- Sugar: 0.2
- Total Carbohydrate: 48.6
- Protein: 7.8
- Saturated Fat: 18.4
- Sodium: 823.9
- Cholesterol: 108.7

348. White Chocolate Chip Macadamia Nut Scones

Serving: 12 serving(s) | Prep: 10mins | Ready in:

Ingredients

- 2 1/2 cups biscuit mix
- 1/4 cup sugar
- 1/4 cup firm butter or 1/4 cup margarine
- 1 cup white chocolate chips
- 1/2 cup chopped macadamia nuts
- 1/4 cup whipping cream (heavy)
- 1 egg

Direction

- Heat oven to 425°F. Spray cookie sheet with cooking spray.
- Stir together biscuit mix and sugar in large bowl. Cut in butter until crumbly. Stir in remaining ingredients.
- Pat dough into 10x7-inch rectangle on cookie sheet (if dough is sticky, dip fingers in the biscuit mix). Cut into 12 rectangles, but don't separate.
- Bake 12 to 14 minutes or until golden brown; carefully separate scones. Serve warm.

Nutrition Information

- Calories: 296.7
- Saturated Fat: 8.1
- Sodium: 367
- Fiber: 1
- Sugar: 15.7
- Protein: 3.9
- Total Fat: 18.7
- Total Carbohydrate: 29.3
- Cholesterol: 37.1

349. Whole Grain Blueberry Ful Muffins

Serving: 13 serving(s) | Prep: 5mins | Ready in:

Ingredients

- 1 1/2 cups whole wheat flour
- 1/2 cup oatmeal
- 1/4 cup sugar
- 1 teaspoon baking powder
- 1/2 teaspoon baking soda
- 1/4 teaspoon salt
- 1 cup nonfat milk (soured with vinegar)
- 1 tablespoon applesauce
- 2 teaspoons canola oil
- 2 egg whites
- 1 cup blueberries (fresh or frozen)

Direction

- Mix dry ingredients in a large bowl.
- Make a well in the center of the mix and add wet ingredients.
- Mix just until combined, then fold in berries.
- Bake 18-20 minutes at 400.

Nutrition Information

- Calories: 96.5
- Cholesterol: 0.4
- Total Carbohydrate: 18.9
- Sodium: 138.3
- Fiber: 2.1
- Sugar: 6.1
- Protein: 3.5
- Total Fat: 1.3
- Saturated Fat: 0.2

350. Whole Grain Fruitcake Muffins

Serving: 12 serving(s) | Prep: 10mins | Ready in:

Ingredients

- 1 cup buttermilk
- 1/3 cup canola oil
- 2 eggs
- 1/3 cup brown sugar
- 1 teaspoon vanilla extract
- 3/4 cup wheat bran

- 1/2 cup rolled oats
- 1 1/4 cups whole wheat flour
- 2 teaspoons cinnamon
- 1/2 teaspoon salt
- 1 tablespoon baking powder
- 1/2 cup candied orange peel (fruitcake mixes)

Direction

- In a medium bowl, mix milk, oil, eggs, brown sugar and vanilla, whisking to combine. Stir in the wheat bran and oats. Allow this to sit for 5 minutes.
- Preheat the oven to 400°F.
- Stir in the flour, cinnamon, salt, and baking powder. Fold in the orange peel.
- Line a 12 cup muffin tin. Distribute the batter between the 12 cups. Bake for about 15 minutes, test them for doneness with a toothpick. Leave the muffins in the pan for 5 minutes. Remove them and cool completely on a wire rack.

Nutrition Information

- Calories: 162.7
- Fiber: 3.6
- Total Carbohydrate: 21.3
- Cholesterol: 36.1
- Protein: 4.6
- Total Fat: 7.7
- Saturated Fat: 0.9
- Sodium: 224.1
- Sugar: 7.1

351. Whole Wheat Banana Flax Muffins

Serving: 12 serving(s) | Prep: 15mins | Ready in:

Ingredients

- 1 1/2 cups whole wheat flour
- 1/2 cup golden flax seed meal
- 1/2 cup quick oats or 1/2 cup quick-cooking barley
- 2 teaspoons baking powder
- 1/2 teaspoon baking soda
- 1 teaspoon cinnamon
- 1/4 teaspoon clove
- 2 ripe mashed bananas
- 2 eggs
- 1 cup almond milk
- 1/4-1/3 cup honey
- 2/3 cup chopped walnuts

Direction

- Preheat oven to 375 degrees.
- Mix flour, flax meal, oats (or barley), baking powder, baking soda, cinnamon and cloves.
- Stir in walnuts.
- Mix eggs, milk, honey and bananas until well combined.
- Stir into dry ingredients.
- Fill muffin cups and bake for about 20 minutes.

Nutrition Information

- Calories: 183.5
- Sodium: 127.7
- Fiber: 4.5
- Cholesterol: 35.2
- Protein: 5.7
- Saturated Fat: 0.9
- Total Carbohydrate: 26.1
- Total Fat: 7.6
- Sugar: 8.6

352. Whole Wheat Cottage Cheese Breakfast Muffins

Serving: 12 muffins | Prep: 10mins | Ready in:

Ingredients

- 2 cups whole wheat flour

- 3/4 cup brown sugar, lightly packed
- 1 teaspoon baking powder
- 1/2 teaspoon baking soda
- 1 pinch salt
- 1 cup 2% fat cottage cheese
- 1/2 cup liquid egg substitute, well shaken
- 2% low-fat milk
- canola oil
- 1 tablespoon lemon zest, finely grated
- lemon juice
- 1 teaspoon vanilla extract
- 1 cup cranberries or 1 cup blueberries
- 1/4 cup almonds, sliced (optional)

Direction

- Preheat oven to 375°F (190°C). Line a 12-cup muffin pan with paper liners. Stir the flour with the sugar, baking powder, baking soda and salt. Whisk the cottage cheese with the eggs, milk, oil, lemon zest, lemon juice and vanilla in a separate bowl. Make a well in the dry ingredients; pour in the wet ingredients and stir just until combined (do not over mix). Fold in the cranberries. Divide the batter evenly between the muffin cups. Sprinkle the tops with almonds (if using).
- Bake for 20 minutes or until golden and a toothpick inserted into the centre of a muffin comes out clean; cool slightly. Serve warm or at room temperature.

Nutrition Information

- Calories: 146.5
- Fiber: 2.6
- Sugar: 14.7
- Total Carbohydrate: 30
- Total Fat: 1
- Saturated Fat: 0.3
- Sodium: 182.1
- Cholesterol: 1.9
- Protein: 5.9

353. Whole Wheat Cranberry Orange Muffins

Serving: 10-12 serving(s) | Prep: 10mins | Ready in:

Ingredients

- 2 cups whole wheat pastry flour
- 2/3 cup sugar substitute (such as Splenda)
- 1 teaspoon baking powder
- 1 teaspoon baking soda
- 1/2 teaspoon salt
- 5 tablespoons butter or 5 tablespoons margarine, melted
- 2/3 cup orange juice, use juice from can of mandarin oranges, adding enough orange juice to make 2/3 cups
- 3 eggs, beaten
- 3/4 cup fresh cranberries
- 1 (11 ounce) can mandarin oranges
- cooking spray

Direction

- Preheat oven to 375°F.
- Combine dry ingredients.
- Melt the butter.
- Whisk the eggs and orange juice into the melted butter.
- Add the liquid to the dry ingredients mixing until just moistened.
- Fold in the cranberries and oranges being careful not to mash the oranges.
- Spoon the batter into a muffin tin that has been coated with cooking spray.
- Bake for 15- 20 minutes, or until firm and golden brown.

Nutrition Information

- Calories: 222.7
- Sodium: 342.5
- Fiber: 3.9
- Cholesterol: 78.7
- Protein: 5.9
- Total Fat: 7.8

- Saturated Fat: 4.2
- Sugar: 14.2
- Total Carbohydrate: 34.4

354. Whole Wheat Honey Flax Biscuits

Serving: 12 biscuits, 12 serving(s) | Prep: 10mins | Ready in:

Ingredients

- 1 1/2 cups whole wheat flour
- 1/4 cup all-purpose flour
- 1/4 cup flax seed meal
- 1 tablespoon baking powder
- 2 tablespoons Smart Balance Omega Plus
- 1 cup buttermilk
- 1/4 cup sugar-free honey

Direction

- Sift dry ingredients together. Cut in Smart Balance with a pastry blender. Add milk and honey, mix quickly.
- Knead dough for a few minutes.
- Divide into 12 portions and place on a lightly oiled baking sheet.
- Bake in a 425°F oven 12 to 15 minutes until lightly browned.

Nutrition Information

- Calories: 95.5
- Total Fat: 3.2
- Sugar: 1.1
- Total Carbohydrate: 14.7
- Cholesterol: 1.3
- Saturated Fat: 0.7
- Sodium: 129.9
- Fiber: 2.3
- Protein: 3.4

355. Whole Wheat Maple Muffins

Serving: 12 serving(s) | Prep: 15mins | Ready in:

Ingredients

- 1/3 cup 2% low-fat milk
- 1 cup plain yogurt
- 1 large egg
- 1/2 cup maple syrup
- 2 cups whole wheat flour
- 1 1/2 teaspoons baking soda
- 1/2 teaspoon cinnamon
- 1/4 teaspoon nutmeg
- 1/2 cup berries (optional)

Direction

- Preheat the oven to 375F and lightly grease a 12-cup muffin tin.
- In a large bowl, whisk together milk, yogurt, egg and maple syrup.
- In a medium bowl, stir together whole wheat pastry flour, baking soda, cinnamon and nutmeg.
- Pour into the large bowl and stir wet and dry ingredients together until just combined, mixing in berries at the last minute, if using.
- Distribute batter evenly in 12 muffin cups.
- Bake for 15-18 minutes at 375F, until the muffin springs back when lightly pressed and a tester comes out clean.
- Remove from tin and cool completely on wire rack before serving.

Nutrition Information

- Calories: 124.5
- Cholesterol: 18.7
- Protein: 4.1
- Total Fat: 1.7
- Saturated Fat: 0.7
- Total Carbohydrate: 24.6
- Sodium: 177.8

- Fiber: 2.2
- Sugar: 9.3

356. Whole Wheat Oat Scones

Serving: 16 scones, 16 serving(s) | Prep: 15mins | Ready in:

Ingredients

- 3/4 cup butter, cold
- 1 cup rolled oats, toasted (old fashioned)
- 2 cups whole wheat flour
- 1 cup all-purpose flour
- 2 tablespoons superfine sugar
- 1 pinch salt
- 2 1/2 teaspoons baking soda
- 2 eggs
- 3/4 cup buttermilk
- 1/3 cup currants

Direction

- Preheat the oven to 400 degrees Fahrenheit. Grease and flour a large baking sheet (I use parchment paper).
- Dice the butter. Mix the dry ingredients in a bowl, then add the butter and rub inches, set aside. In another bowl whisk together the eggs and buttermilk. Set aside 2 tablespoons for glazing.
- Stir the remaining egg mixture into the dry ingredients to form a dough. Stir in the currants.
- Roll out the dough on a lightly floured surface to about 3/4 inch thick. Stamp out rounds with a floured cutter. Place on the prepared baking sheet and brush with the reserved egg mixture.
- Bake for 12-15 minutes until golden brown. Leave to cool slightly before serving.

Nutrition Information

- Calories: 203.4
- Sodium: 289.8
- Protein: 5
- Cholesterol: 49.8
- Total Fat: 10
- Saturated Fat: 5.8
- Fiber: 2.7
- Sugar: 4.3
- Total Carbohydrate: 24.6

357. Ww 1 Pt. Weight Watcher Muffins

Serving: 18 muffins | Prep: 5mins | Ready in:

Ingredients

- 3 cups fiber one all-bran cereal
- 1 (19 ounce) boxkrusteaz fat-free blueberry muffin mix
- 2 1/2 cups hot water
- 1 1/2 teaspoons baking powder

Direction

- Mix All-Bran w/hot water.
- Stir and set aside.
- Add baking powder to the Krusteaz mix.
- Mix all together.
- Bake according to muffin box.

Nutrition Information

- Calories: 27.1
- Protein: 1.4
- Total Fat: 0.5
- Saturated Fat: 0.1
- Sugar: 1.6
- Total Carbohydrate: 7.8
- Cholesterol: 0
- Sodium: 58.1
- Fiber: 3

358. Ww Instant Oatmeal Muffins (1 Ww Point Each)

Serving: 6 muffins, 6 serving(s) | Prep: 5mins | Ready in:

Ingredients

- 1 (1 1/2 ounce) packet instant oatmeal, any flavor (I used maple and brown sugar)
- 1/4 cup flour
- 1 teaspoon baking powder
- 1/4 cup sweetened applesauce
- 2 -3 ounces diet soda, any flavor
- 6 teaspoons light brown sugar

Direction

- Mix first 5 ingredients.
- Spoon into 6 muffin cups.
- Sprinkle top of each muffin with 1 teaspoons brown sugar.
- Bake at 375 for 15-20 minutes.

Nutrition Information

- Calories: 70.3
- Protein: 1.5
- Total Fat: 0.6
- Sodium: 65.1
- Total Carbohydrate: 15.4
- Cholesterol: 0
- Saturated Fat: 0.1
- Fiber: 0.9
- Sugar: 4.6

359. Yo Yo Biscuits

Serving: 12 biscuits | Prep: 15mins | Ready in:

Ingredients

- For biscuits
- 185 g butter, softened
- 75 g icing sugar
- 225 g plain flour
- 75 g custard powder or 75 g cornstarch
- 1 teaspoon vanilla extract
- For butter cream
- 130 g butter, softened
- 165 g icing sugar
- 1 teaspoon lemon juice
- 1 teaspoon lemon zest

Direction

- Preheat oven to 170°C.
- Cream butter and icing sugar until light. Add sifted flour and custard powder. Mix well until forms into smooth dough.
- Roll dough into logs and cut it up into small pieces, same size about 30g each. You should have about 24 pieces.
- Form into balls and place on tray and press with a fork.
- Bake for about 15 minutes. They should be very pale almost no color.
- Tip: Don't over bake them they will be dry.
- For butter-cream:
- With electric mixer whip the softened butter with icing sugar until light and fluffy. Add lemon juice and zest and more or less up to your taste.
- When biscuits are cooled join together with butter cream.
- Tip: If you prefer chocolate butter cream omit lemon juice and zest and add 2 tablespoons cocoa powder and 1tsp. vanilla extract.

Nutrition Information

- Calories: 351.4
- Sodium: 187.2
- Sugar: 19.7
- Cholesterol: 56.1
- Protein: 2.6
- Total Carbohydrate: 38
- Total Fat: 21.4
- Saturated Fat: 13.4
- Fiber: 0.7

360. Yoghurt Corn Muffins With Corn

Serving: 6 big muffins | Prep: 10mins | Ready in:

Ingredients

- 125 g fine polenta or 125 g cornmeal
- 55 g flour (I use spelt)
- 70 g whole wheat flour (I use spelt)
- 1/4 teaspoon baking soda
- 1 teaspoon baking powder
- 1 tablespoon sugar (more if you like it sweeter)
- 125 g yoghurt
- 1/4 cup water, about
- 1 egg, beaten
- 200 g corn kernels (I use canned)
- 125 g cheese, shredded (optional)

Direction

- In a big bowl combine all of the dry ingredients (polenta through to sugar) and mix well. Make a well in the centre.
- In a separate bowl combine yoghurt and egg. Add corn kernels, water and cheese if using. Mix well and pour into the well in the dry ingredients. Mix to form a soft, thick dough. If it is too dry, add more water by tbsp. until your dough looks right (it should be creamy and thick, very much like cake dough).
- Pour into prepared muffin tins.
- Bake in the preheated oven at 200°C/400°F for 15-20 minutes or until lightly golden and baked through.
- Enjoy!

Nutrition Information

- Calories: 240.5
- Total Fat: 3.1
- Sodium: 144.4
- Cholesterol: 33.7
- Protein: 8
- Saturated Fat: 0.9
- Fiber: 4.6
- Sugar: 3.3
- Total Carbohydrate: 48.6

361. Yogurt Banana Muffins

Serving: 96 mini-muffins, 24 serving(s) | Prep: 10mins | Ready in:

Ingredients

- 1 1/4 cups sugar
- 1/2 cup butter or 1/2 cup margarine, softened
- 2 large eggs
- 3 large bananas, mashed (or 4, to taste)
- 1 (6 ounce) container vanilla yogurt (or plain Greek yogurt and 1 t vanilla)
- 2 1/2 cups all-purpose flour
- 1 teaspoon baking soda
- 1 teaspoon salt
- 1 cup semi-sweet chocolate chips (optional)

Direction

- Preheat oven to 350, placing rack in lowest position.
- Prepare mini-muffin tins with paper liners.
- Cream sugar and butter in large bowl.
- Mix in eggs with mixer until well blended.
- Add bananas and yogurt, and beat until smooth.
- Add baking soda and salt. Mix.
- Fold in flour until it's all moistened.
- Stir in chips.
- Fill liners in pan about 3/4 of the way. I use a cookie scoop and they go quickly and turn out uniform.
- Bake 20 minutes on bottom rack.

Nutrition Information

- Calories: 147.1

- Total Fat: 4.7
- Sodium: 192.8
- Cholesterol: 26.6
- Protein: 2.3
- Saturated Fat: 2.8
- Fiber: 0.8
- Sugar: 12.9
- Total Carbohydrate: 24.6

362. Yummy Chocolate Pumpkin Muffins

Serving: 12 muffins | Prep: 5mins | Ready in:

Ingredients

- 1 (18 ounce) box chocolate cake mix
- 1 (15 ounce) can pumpkin puree
- 1/2-3/4 cup water
- white frosting (optional)

Direction

- Preheat the oven to 400 degrees.
- Put cake mix in a large bowl.
- In a separate bowl, mix 1/2 cup water with pumpkin puree.
- Slowly stir in pumpkin mixture to cake mix. Add more water if batter is too thick. (HINT it should be thicker than normal cake batter).
- Line muffin cups and fill 3/4 with batter.
- Bake according to cake box directions.
- Top with optional frosting when cool.

Nutrition Information

- Calories: 191.3
- Sodium: 351.4
- Fiber: 1.2
- Sugar: 16.8
- Total Carbohydrate: 33.4
- Cholesterol: 0
- Total Fat: 6.7
- Saturated Fat: 1.4
- Protein: 2.9

363. Yummy Healthy Muffins

Serving: 6 muffins, 6 serving(s) | Prep: 10mins | Ready in:

Ingredients

- 3/4 cup whole wheat flour
- 2 teaspoons baking powder
- 1/2 teaspoon baking soda
- 1 teaspoon cinnamon
- 1 scoop vanilla protein powder
- 1/3 cup soymilk
- 1 egg
- 1/4 cup canola oil
- 2 carrots
- 1 cup oatmeal
- 1/4 cup raisins

Direction

- Mix together all wet ingredients.
- Mix all dry, except oatmeal and raisins, in a separate bowl.
- Add dry to wet.
- Add oatmeal and raisins.
- Bake at 400F for 12 minute.

Nutrition Information

- Calories: 230.5
- Protein: 6.3
- Total Fat: 11.4
- Saturated Fat: 1.1
- Sodium: 261.1
- Fiber: 4.3
- Total Carbohydrate: 28.1
- Sugar: 4.9
- Cholesterol: 35.2

364. Zucchini Lemon Muffins

Serving: 12 serving(s) | Prep: 10mins | Ready in:

Ingredients

- 2 1/4 cups all-purpose flour
- 1/2 cup granulated sugar
- 2 teaspoons double-acting baking powder
- 1 teaspoon baking soda
- 1 1/2 cups shredded zucchini
- 3/4 cup thawed frozen egg substitute
- 1/8 cup vegetable oil
- 1/8 cup unsweetened applesauce
- 1 teaspoon grated lemon, rind of

Direction

- Preheat oven to 350 degrees.
- Line twelve 2.
- 5 inch muffin-pan cups with paper baking cups; set aside.
- In large mixing bowl combine flour, sugar, baking powder, and baking soda set aside.
- In medium mixing bowl, combine remaining ingredients, stirring to combine; add to flour mixture and stir until moistened (do not over mix).
- Fill each baking cup with an equal amount of batter (each will be in about 2/3 full).
- Bake in middle of center comes out dry.
- Remove muffins from pan to wire rack and let cool.

Nutrition Information

- Calories: 154.9
- Saturated Fat: 0.4
- Fiber: 0.8
- Total Carbohydrate: 27.4
- Cholesterol: 0.2
- Protein: 4.5
- Total Fat: 3
- Sugar: 8.8
- Sodium: 216

365. Ice Cream Muffins

Serving: 12 muffins | Prep: 10mins | Ready in:

Ingredients

- 2 cups self raising flour (very important)
- 2 cups ice cream (the better quality the ice cream the better quality muffin in the end)

Direction

- Measure 2 cups ice cream and allow to soften.
- Add to 2 cups of flour and stir until mixed.
- Spoon into paper muffin cups and bake in 375 oven approx. 15-18 minutes.
- I know this sounds crazy but they really work!
- REMEMBER the better ice cream gives a better product. My first batch was with generic vanilla, they were o.k. but not as good as the higher quality ice creams.

Nutrition Information

- Calories: 124.1
- Fiber: 0.7
- Total Carbohydrate: 21.6
- Protein: 3
- Total Fat: 2.8
- Sodium: 19.6
- Sugar: 5.2
- Cholesterol: 10.6
- Saturated Fat: 1.7

Index

A

Almond 3,11,12

Apple 3,4,5,6,7,11,12,13,14,15,16,70,84,108,116,117,119,126,138,151,154,155,185

Apricot 3,4,5,6,16,87,105,150

B

Bacon 3,4,6,33,86,116,156

Baking 3,6,19,20,27,102,145,160,187

Banana 3,4,5,6,7,19,20,21,22,23,24,25,28,29,30,69,72,76,78,88,89,103,113,114,119,127,131,135,137,140,145,146,154,161,166,168,169,170,173,174,191,196

Basil 4,61

Beef 3,28

Berry 4,90,92

Biscuits 3,4,5,6,7,9,18,20,28,31,33,41,48,49,53,54,59,62,63,65,66,67,70,71,73,74,75,76,80,83,85,96,99,102,103,104,105,106,107,118,121,126,133,136,138,142,145,158,160,163,165,167,172,173,178,182,184,187,189,193,195

Blackberry 3,34

Blueberry 3,4,5,6,7,17,35,36,37,60,62,79,83,90,91,97,115,118,120,121,123,137,139,159,170,173,183,190

Bran 3,4,5,6,7,9,15,16,23,24,28,37,38,44,45,46,63,91,96,100,115,119,121,122,124,125,132,133,138,139,140,144,145,147,151,154,169,174,179,180,194

Bread 1,3,4,5,6,8,27,65,78,119,145,157,168

Buns 3,31

Butter 3,5,6,40,41,46,94,106,116,142,144,145,147,148,150,154,160,165,180,189

C

Cake 8

Caramel 3,43

Carrot 3,4,5,6,7,26,27,43,44,45,46,93,126,130,158,186

Cheddar 3,4,5,6,16,31,34,47,48,54,62,101,102,103,156

Cheese 3,4,5,6,7,28,29,35,48,50,54,62,73,86,92,105,162,163,164,167,175,178,182,183,188,191

Cherry 6,150

Chipotle 4,50

Chocolate 3,4,5,6,7,8,19,22,24,51,52,53,54,89,92,103,113,144,148,185,189,197

Cinnamon 3,4,5,6,7,15,21,33,54,55,56,128,146,177,181

Cocktail 3,48

Coconut 4,5,6,7,58,110,161,179

Coffee 4,58,59

Cranberry 4,5,6,7,64,65,78,109,141,164,179,192

Cream 3,5,6,7,15,18,24,48,53,77,82,83,85,100,105,108,119,127,129,132,137,141,158,175,189,195,196,198

Crumble 5,6,116,152

Custard 4,66

D

Date 3,4,12,27,45,68

Dill 5,101

E

Egg 3,4,5,6,10,12,30,67,79,86,116,135,152,163,186

English muffin 86,162,163,183,188

F

Fat
3,4,5,6,7,8,9,10,11,12,13,14,15,16,17,18,19,20,21,22,23,24,25,26,27,28,29,30,31,32,33,34,35,36,37,38,39,40,41,42,43,44,45,46,47,48,49,50,51,52,53,54,55,56,57,58,59,60,61,62,63,64,65,66,67,68,69,70,71,72,73,74,75,76,77,78,79,80,81,82,83,84,85,86,87,88,89,90,91,92,93,94,95,96,97,98,99,100,101,102,103,104,105,106,107,108,109,110,111,112,113,114,115,116,117,118,119,120,121,122,123,124,125,126,127,128,129,130,131,132,133,134,135,136,137,138,139,140,141,142,143,144,145,146,147,148,149,150,151,152,153,154,155,156,157,158,159,160,161,162,163,164,165,166,167,168,169,170,171,172,173,174,175,176,177,178,179,180,181,182,183,184,185,186,187,188,189,190,191,192,193,194,195,196,197,198

Flour 3,4,11,19,56,58,123,187

French bread 75

Fruit 3,4,7,10,31,72,81,190

G

Garlic 5,6,54,103,160,165

Gin 3,4,5,7,22,27,82,83,93,97,105,108,128,129,186

Grain 5,7,135,190

H

Ham 4,5,86,126

Heart 5,120

Honey 3,5,6,7,17,99,100,150,180,193

I

Icing 8,81,96,97,109

J

Jelly 5,6,104,142

Jus 9,74,80,84,110

L

Lemon 3,5,7,37,108,109,110,111,112,123,198

M

Macadamia 7,189

Mango 5,111,130

Molasses 4,82

Muffins
3,4,5,6,7,8,9,10,11,12,13,14,15,16,17,19,21,22,23,24,25,26,27,28,29,30,32,35,36,37,38,39,40,42,43,44,45,46,49,50,51,52,53,54,55,58,59,60,61,62,63,64,65,66,67,68,69,70,71,72,73,77,78,79,81,82,84,86,87,88,89,90,91,92,93,94,95,96,97,100,103,104,106,107,108,110,111,112,113,114,115,116,117,118,119,121,122,124,125,126,127,128,129,130,131,132,133,134,135,136,137,138,139,140,141,142,143,144,145,147,148,149,150,151,152,153,154,155,156,158,159,161,162,163,164,166,168,169,170,171,172,173,174,175,176,177,178,179,180,182,183,185,186,188,190,191,192,193,194,195,196,197,198

Mushroom 5,135

N

Nectarine 7,180

Nut
3,4,7,8,9,10,11,12,13,14,15,16,17,18,19,20,21,22,23,24,25,26,27,28,29,30,31,32,33,34,35,36,37,38,39,40,41,42,43,44,45,46,47,48,49,50,51,52,53,54,55,56,57,58,59,60,61,62,63,64,65,66,67,68,69,70,71,72,73,74,75,76,77,78,79,80,81,82,83,84,85,86,87,88,89,90,91,92,93,94,95,96,97,98,99,100,101,102,103,104,105,106,107,108,109,110,111,112,113,114,115,116,117,118,119,120,121,122,123,124,125,126,127,128,129,130,131,132,133,134,135,136,137,138,139,140,141,142,143,144,145,146,147,148,149,150,151,152,153,154,155,156,157,158,159,160,161,162,163,164,165,166,167,168,169,170,171,172,173,174,175,176,177,178,179,180,181,182,183,184,185,186,187,188,189,190,191,192,193,194,195,196,197,198

O

Oatcakes 3,4,48,57

Oatmeal 3,4,5,6,7,30,38,76,94,95,113,117,122,140,141,142,143,153,159,195

Oil 6,44,55,117,144,146

Onion 4,7,54,74,178,182

Orange 3,4,5,6,7,42,65,78,119,122,147,150,174,176,192

P

Pancakes 6,166

Parmesan 34,102,162

Peach 5,7,100,180

Pear 4,6,7,72,148,181

Pecan 3,13,48

Peel 155

Pepper 3,7,33,102,181

Pineapple 3,4,6,43,68,86,149

Pistachio 3,6,17,150,185

Pizza 4,7,86,188

Port 110

Potato 3,6,39,47,149

Praline 3,25

Prune 5,94

Pulse 45,123,138

Pumpkin 3,5,6,7,32,107,117,122,151,152,153,154,157,168,197

R

Raspberry 3,4,5,46,58,117

Rhubarb 5,6,112,177

Rice 5,6,100,159,176

Rosemary 6,7,34,160,187

Rum 6,160

S

Sage 6,165

Salad 6,161

Salmon 6,161

Salt 145

Sausage 4,6,86,162,163

Savory 6,163,164,165

Seeds 6,157

Soda 145

Soup 6,171

Spices 67

Spinach 5,116

Squash 5,94

Strawberry 6,174,175,176

Sugar 4,5,6,8,9,10,11,12,13,14,15,16,17,18,19,20,21,22,23,24,25,26,27,28,29,30,31,32,33,34,35,36,37,38,39,40,41,42,43,44,45,46,47,48,49,50,51,52,53,54,55,56,57,58,59,60,61,62,63,64,65,66,67,68,69,70,71,72,73,74,75,76,77,78,79,80,81,82,83,84,85,86,87,88,89,90,91,92,93,94,95,96,97,98,99,100,101,102,103,104,105,106,107,108,109,110,111,112,113,114,115,116,117,118,119,120,121,122,123,124,125,126,127,128,129,130,131,132,133,134,135,136,137,138,139,140,141,142,143,144,145,146,147,148,149,150,151,152,153,154,155,156,157,158,159,160,161,162,163,164,165,166,167,168,169,170,171,172,173,174,175,176,177,178,179,180,181,182,183,184,185,186,187,188,189,190,191,192,193,194,195,196,197,198

T

Tarragon 3,47

Tea 3,7,31,181

Tomato 4,7,80,178,187

V

Vegan 3,5,6,7,15,112,126,157,185,186,187

Vegetarian 7,188

W

Walnut 3,4,6,21,64,87,136

Y

Yoghurt 7,196

Z

Zest 123

Conclusion

Thank you again for downloading this book!

I hope you enjoyed reading about my book!

If you enjoyed this book, please take the time to share your thoughts and post a review on Amazon. It'd be greatly appreciated!

Write me an honest review about the book – I truly value your opinion and thoughts and I will incorporate them into my next book, which is already underway.

Thank you!

If you have any questions, **feel free to contact at:** author@jumbocookbook.com

Vicky Johnson

jumbocookbook.com

Made in United States
Orlando, FL
20 February 2024